REDESIGNING

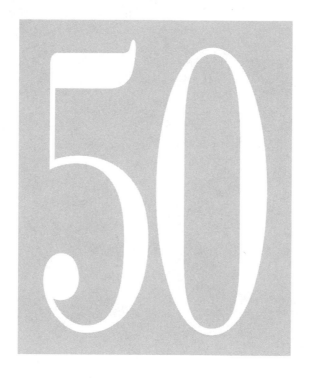

Also by Oz Garcia

THE BALANCE

LOOK AND FEEL FABULOUS FOREVER

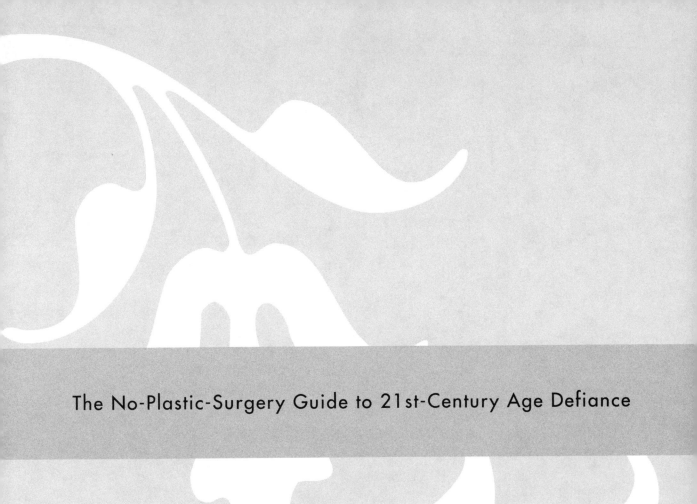

The No-Plastic-Surgery Guide to 21st-Century Age Defiance

REDESIGNING

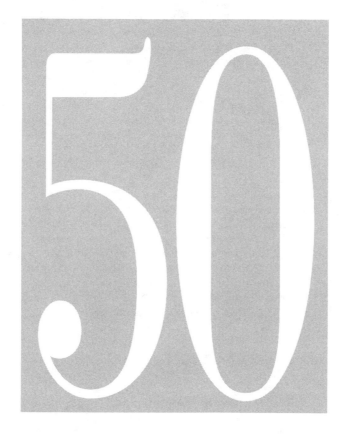

OZ GARCIA

WITH SHARYN KOLBERG

Collins

An Imprint of HarperCollins *Publishers*

REDESIGNING 50. Copyright © 2008 by Oz Garcia. All rights reserved. Printed in the United States of America. No part of this book may be used or reproduced in any manner whatsoever without written permission except in the case of brief quotations embodied in critical articles and reviews. For information, address HarperCollins Publishers, 10 East 53rd Street, New York, NY 10022.

HarperCollins books may be purchased for educational, business, or sales promotional use. For information, please write: Special Markets Department, HarperCollins Publishers, 10 East 53rd Street, New York, NY 10022.

FIRST EDITION

Designed by Ellen Cipriano

Library of Congress Cataloging-in-Publication Data

Garcia, Oz.
    Redesigning 50 : the no plastic surgery guide to 21st-century age defiance / Oz Garcia, with Sharyn Kolberg.
        p. cm.
    ISBN-13: 978-0-06-076047-2
    1. Nutrition. 2. Diet. 3. Health. 4. Exercise. 5. Beauty, Personal. 6. Face—Care and hygiene. I. Title. II. Title: Redesigning fifty.

RA784.G358 2007
613.7—dc22

2006051816

08   09   10   11   12   WBT/RRD   9   8   7   6   5   4   3   2   1

This book is dedicated to my mother and father,
Clara and Osvaldo Garcia.
In loving memory of my father,
with a special message:
I know how proud you would be, Dad.
Love, Oz.

CONTENTS

PART III BEAUTY:

Facing Up to Aging   83

PART IV ALCHEMY:

Exploring the Biological Landscape of Age Reversal   129

ACKNOWLEDGMENTS

My gratitude and acknowledgments go to a great number of people. For many reasons, this book was a long time in the making, and I thank everyone involved for their perseverance and patience. I especially want to thank Mary Ellen O'Neill and everyone at HarperCollins for continuing to believe in this project.

Thanks also to

The unbelievable Laura Powers, my vice president: Without her, nothing would get done. She is the central source of ideas and gravity for this project, and for much of my life.

Sharyn Kolberg, who infused her great craft and worked with me at every corner of this book to make it a highly informative and enjoyable read—as she has done with all of my books.

Tony Colletti and Gerardo Somoza for all their hard work, dedication, and friendship.

Anna Bliss and Toni Sciarra, my editors, whose insightful thoughts and tenacious grip have allowed this project to move forward efficiently and achieve its highest aspiration.

Judith Regan, my eternal gratitude for everything she did for this project.

All the diverse groups of experts—from the culinary artists to medical professionals and everyone in between. Their contributions will be apparent to readers in the extraordinary interviews throughout the book.

Albert and Claudia Garcia. My brother, Albert, is my partner for life and the backbone of all our work.

Judy Taylor and Jenny Fisherman-Ruff for their support: they are a wonderful public relations team.

In addition, a thank-you to my extended family of staff, friends, and partners: Tara Santiago, Deirdre Mahony, Liz Belson, John Aslanian, Randy and Hayley Corwick, and everyone at Restore Spa. Thanks as well to Mila Jouravleva, my European partner, and Bijan Khezri. Thanks also to Barbara Ligeti and everyone at Lime TV and Gaiam.

INTRODUCING
THE NEW 50

"How old would you be if you didn't know how old you was?"
—SATCHEL PAIGE,
BASEBALL HALL OF FAMER

Are you fifty or thereabouts? Chances are you don't look, act, or feel the way your parents did at fifty. It's a whole new era in the art and science of aging, and that's what this book is about: redesigning the rest of your life to slow down your biological clock and keep you looking and feeling as young as possible for as long as possible. It's also about redefining what it means to get chronologically older even as you keep the energy, vitality, and appearance of youth.

This book is about *healthy* aging—staying active physically and mentally, looking your best whatever your age, and knowing what you need to keep yourself in the best possible shape for years to come. So welcome to *Redesigning 50*. In this book, we're going to introduce you to what fifty looks like in the twenty-first century and help you take advantage of the finest that science and artistry have to offer to make "middle age" the best it's ever been, without going under the knife. Although plastic surgery might be appropriate for some people in certain circumstances, there are now many far more enlightened antiaging options to bring you to what I like to call the New 50: a fitter, healthier, better-looking middle age than you ever imagined possible.

Do we even know what middle age means anymore? If you're anywhere near the age of fifty, you probably remember that the mantra of the 1960s was "Don't trust anyone over the age of thirty." When we were teenagers, we thought that thirty marked the beginning of middle age. I know I did. But now, having passed the thirty-year marker many years ago, I'm no longer sure how to define middle age. Old definitions no longer apply. Middle-aged women are now having babies. Men and women in their sixties and seventies are climbing mountains, traveling into outer space, and making greater achievements than are many of their more youthful counterparts. In today's world, middle age is no longer a stage of life to be dreaded or feared, but one that we can fully enjoy and embrace.

Aging takes most of us by surprise. We look in the mirror one day, or get up out of a chair, or try to do something we used to do effortlessly—and suddenly we realize that we've actually gotten older. That's what happened to me. Even though I don't always want to admit it, I have started to experience the universal signs of reaching a certain . . . maturity. I need reading glasses. I can't run at the same pace or with the same stamina I used to. It's become a little more difficult to regulate my weight.

I've started to ask myself questions. What can I do now and for the rest of my life to make the coming years as good as those that have passed? Do I need to worry about health concerns that some have called the diseases of aging? And how do I not only remain healthy but feel good—and look good, too?

Fortunately, I have a privileged perspective from which to explore and answer these concerns. For the past twenty years, I've been a successful nutritional consultant in New York City, the head of health and nutritional services for Equinox Fitness Clubs worldwide, a consultant to the East Coast Alliance of Trainers and to the world-renowned Life Extension Foundation, and the author of *The Balance* and *Look and Feel Fabulous Forever*. Over the course of my professional and personal experience, I've come to grasp the true importance of everything from managing our hormones to how much sleep we get (yes, we really do need eight hours) to the most advanced diagnostic testing available today to gauge every aspect of our health, and the full range of products we can now put to use.

Using the latest information and most innovative means available, I aim to help you experience the highest levels of well-being so that you can be more productive, have better relationships, reduce needless suffering, manage your moods, reduce the use of medication when appropriate, and overcome infirmity more quickly. Ultimately, I want you to stay in the game as long as possible, playing at peak performance.

I'm not foolish enough to promise that you won't get old, but I am saying that antiaging techniques have come a long, long way in recent years. I'm not saying you can stop all deterioration of the body as you get older, but I am saying you can lay down speed bumps to slow the process and in many ways even reverse the signs and symptoms of aging.

Middle age represents more than a number; it marks a hormonal shift that appears as menopause in women and andropause in men. Even if our appearance doesn't give away our age, our hormones do. Some people feel that these hormonal shifts mean the end of their youth and vitality. I'm here to say that this is just not true and that with the knowledge and scientific advances we have today, middle age can be the best part of your life. You *can* modify your diet and lifestyle to lead a longer, happier, and healthier life. You *can* have a vibrant sex life. You *can* reduce and even reverse much of the damage done to your skin from dietary and environmental abuse. You *can* look and feel young again.

The best part is that you can achieve all this without having to live in a dietary bubble. You will learn how to make healthy choices and still enjoy food in a nonrestrictive manner—both at home and while dining out, whether it's at a mainstream restaurant like Gennaro Sbarro's or at a four-star restaurant with a chef like David Bouley.

You will get some really sound pointers on the functional effects of particular foods. You'll learn not just which foods are good for you and why, but also what gives them their rejuvenating properties. As we age, we get immunologically weaker; changes in our genetic expression cause us to be prone to diabetes, heart disease, and excitotoxic damage to our brains (excitotoxins are food additives like MSG and aspartame, which can literally stimulate neurons to death). Food can be a critical tool in protecting us against the tectonic shifts that occur within our bodies as we get older.

You will learn that fitness is extremely critical as we age, not only to maintain physical strength and muscle mass but also to keep our minds sharp and efficient. For this book, I have consulted with some of the top experts in the fields of mind and body fitness for people in their forties, fifties, and beyond.

You will also learn that managing stress becomes more important as we age. Things that were once seen as far out (such as yoga and meditation) or self-indulgent (such as massage and the spa experience) have now been proved to be major components of longer, healthier lives. I will help you understand what stress is, and how you can regulate and reduce it.

The main reason I wrote this book was to identify the key elements in redefining this midpoint in our lives. Being fifty (and beyond) today means living in an option-filled environment. There are so many things you can do to maintain the state of good health and well-being described in this book simply by following certain protocols laid out here. These steps are not radical. As you will see from reading this book, in every field there are various points of view, so you can choose which may be best for you, your circumstances, and your lifestyle. But each one gives you a barometer, a means by which you can gauge how you are doing now, what you can do going forward, how you can erase years of wear and tear on your body, and how you can prevent damage in the future.

It isn't that I want you to be fifty years old and look as if you're twenty. I want you to be fifty years old and have your body respond as if you were a fit and healthy thirty-five-year-old. I want you to be able to spend the next fifty years able to regulate the speed at which you're aging by how you use food, supplements, and nutraceuticals; how you manage stress; how you incorporate fitness and exercise into your life; and how you take care of and maintain your youthful appearance.

The goal of this book is to present you with options. I have mined the knowledge of health professionals in both traditional and alternative medicine to present the best of what's available for the "boomer" population. These professionals are at the top of their fields; I have worked with many of them and greatly admire their practices. They are all extremely smart, caring professionals who share my philosophy of health: to help people attain and maintain active, vital lifestyles for as long as possible by combining the best of conventional medicine with the newest discoveries in health care.

While I have cast a broad net to cover the major non–plastic-surgery components of antiaging, and consulted professionals from many health and beauty fields, far more options and professional services are available to boomers in this country than any single book could contain. We are very fortunate in that respect, but this plethora of choices has its downside as well. How do you know what's best for you? How do you choose one viewpoint over another? That's one of the reasons I wrote this book—to introduce you to some of the options you will find as you enter this new era of age reversal and to provide you with a preliminary information guide. In this book you may find suggestions, techniques, and methodologies that you have never heard of or considered before. I don't expect that you will try them all. I do encourage you to explore the areas that interest you and to find the methods that work best for your lifestyle and circumstances.

From a Living Perspective

Obviously, a great deal of information (much of it conflicting) can be obtained through books and on the Internet. What's usually missing from these kinds of sources, however, is the human perspective. What does it mean for a real person to complete a detoxifying/cleansing regimen, get diagnostic testing, go to a cosmetic dentist, undergo physical therapy, visit a dermatologist, practice yoga, or go to a spa?

The only way I can help you understand this kind of journey is to present you with real people who have gone through these processes. Throughout the chapters ahead, you will find quotes and interviews from people who have visited the kinds of specialists and health professionals introduced in this book, who have gone through testing, followed exercise regimens, and taken yoga classes—in other words, who, like everyone else who lives in the real world, have struggled to find the time and energy to make healthy changes in their lives.

So welcome to *Redesigning 50*, which will send you into the next several decades of your life with much of the knowledge and inspiration you'll need

TURNING BACK THE
CLOCK WITH OZ

I'm fifty-four years old, and I met Oz when I was forty-four. I now feel as if I've gone from fifty-four to thirty-four. When I first met him, I had hit the wall. I was running six miles a day, and all of a sudden I was exhausted. I was falling asleep every day at three in the afternoon. I went to see Oz because he was recommended by a friend. To say I was skeptical is an understatement. I told him up front: "I'm not going to take any of your stupid vitamins. I'm not going to listen to anything you have to say. But what do you have to say?"

He told me that my adrenals were exhausted and that I needed to change my eating habits. I thought I had a good diet. I ate a lot of fish and salads. He said that I needed to do a cleanse and get my liver straightened out.

I followed a detox program for about a week. By the fifth or sixth day, I was flying. I was back up and running, and I've never stopped. Now I'm up early in the morning and up until eleven at night.

He said I needed to make sure I was off all caffeine. He was very strict. He said, "If you don't get off the caffeine, I don't even want to see you again." I said, "You're out of your mind. It's probably Lyme disease." I went and got tested. I got tested twice. It wasn't Lyme disease. Finally I said, "Okay, fine; I'll listen to you."

For me, the coffee was a detriment. It was really hurting me, and I didn't even know it. I didn't even think I was drinking that much. But Oz asked me to keep a food log and to write down everything I was eating and drinking. I showed it to him and said, "You see, I don't drink coffee." He said, "What's that?" I said "That's the cup I have when I get up in the morning to get me going." "What's that?" he asked. "That's the one cup after breakfast." He said, "What's that?" "That's the late-morning pick-me-up cup." "What's that?" "That's the one after lunch." "What's that?" "That's the one at four in the afternoon when I'm really tired." "What's that?" "That's the one after dinner." He said, "That's six cups a day! Of course you're a coffee drinker." I had no idea.

Working with Oz is a learning process. He helps you become a good detective about your own health. He helps you learn to take care of yourself. He always takes a sensible approach. It's not extreme like Atkins or Pritikin. It's his own way. He's been a wealth of information and a wealth of knowledge.

In some ways I'm unique, because I have a chronic disease that can be very debilitating. Some people end up in the hospital. I take care of myself, and I feel great. I'm involved in several different businesses, I run around, I play. If anything, my problem is that sometimes I think I'm too young. I have to remember that I'm a little bit older now.

Oz taught me to be self-sufficient. He took me beyond healthy. He took me to a point where ten years later I feel ten years younger than when I started.

I am, however, a human being, so sometimes I'll call him up in the middle of February and say, "I don't know what's going on. I have headaches, and I'm tired." He says, "What are you doing? Let me guess. You're eating ice cream and chocolate and peanuts. Cut that stuff out." Sure enough, the headaches go away.

He always teaches that everyone's got a margin for error. He doesn't tell anyone what to do. If I ask him, "Can I drink alcohol?" he says, "If you can have one or two glasses of wine, great. But if you're the type of person who can't tolerate alcohol, then learn to recognize that about yourself. You have a smaller margin of error in that area." He basically teaches you to be the owner of your own body and to educate yourself about your own margins for error.

JOHN ASLANIAN, FIFTY-FOUR,
MEDICAL MANAGEMENT CONSULTANT

to make them as vibrant, productive, and happy as possible. The people you'll meet in this book have revolutionized their health and their habits to erase many years from the aging process, and so can you. Let the journey begin.

FOOD:

FUELING YOURSELF TO A YOUNGER BODY

A S A NUTRITIONIST, I've found that my thoughts about food have evolved over the years. When I wrote *The Balance*, I was thinking of using food in terms of correcting individual metabolic imbalances. When I wrote *Look and Feel Fabulous Forever*, I introduced the Paleo-tech diet, which was based on our ancestral and historical ways of eating (and the fact that we are organic bodies not evolved to eat large portions of processed foods).

We were designed by nature to have a voracious appetite. This was useful in a different time, when we had to hunt and gather our food. We have the primal instincts of an animal that's always on the prowl for food, in a present-day dietary landscape where food is all too easily accessible and all too unhealthy. Much of what we eat in the modern world is unrecognizable by our bodies in terms of what would enhance our health. We've woven ourselves a tangled web, and we must fight our way out. As Natalie Angier stated in an article titled

"'Hunger': Never Enough" that appeared in the *New York Times* on September 18, 2005: "That we have deep-seated and contradictory feelings about our appetites is undeniable. That hunger for food can be a force more powerful than reason, common decency or love itself even overfed Westerners can believe. As a scientist once said to me, 'Most of us are only nine meals away from murder.'"

In this country, we have become so obsessed with food—or, more specifically, with dieting (if we're not on a diet, we think we should be)—that we have lost nearly all the enjoyment that food can bring to our lives. Food is delicious, food is beautiful, food is sustenance, food is life. Yet we now have such a complex relationship with food that we can't sit down to a meal without having our heads spin. It's time to change the way we think about food.

ONE

OZ EATS HIS WORDS

REDESIGNING THE WAY WE EAT

WE ALL NEED to move toward a more mature relationship with food. If we want to be healthy, we need to move away from what I believe is a uniquely American experiment: "dieting by extremes"—that is, eating food cooked only one way (or not cooked at all) or eliminating entire food groups. The goal of the *Redesigning 50* eating program is to help you establish a natural, comfortable relationship with food that allows you to eat a great variety of proteins and carbohydrates, cooked in ways that are delicious as well as nutritionally sound.

Ironically, I came to these conclusions about the American diet when I left the country. In other parts of the world, I learned not only about the foods of other countries but also about their mealtime traditions. Specifically, I visited two areas of the world with very different foods on their menus; yet, I also found some striking similarities. Both countries have a noticeable lack of overweight people. Both countries have long-standing and continuing traditions of family mealtimes. And in both countries, meals often consist of many different courses served over a period of two to three hours.

The two countries I visited were Japan and Greece.

Melding Traditions

I spent several weeks in Japan recently and decided that while I was there, I would eat only traditional Japanese foods. Almost all the social occasions and business meetings took place around food. I became enchanted with the Japanese diet not only because of its nutritional content but also because of its beautiful presentation. Even on the subway in Tokyo, you can get a lunchtime Bento box (single-portion takeout meal) with a bit of fish in one compartment, chicken in another, some rice, seaweed, and pickled vegetables. The meal is both filling and aesthetically pleasing. When my hosts took me to a traditional restaurant in Kyoto, our business lunch lasted almost three hours. We were served many courses; each course was small in portion, but rich in flavor and centered on vegetables.

I've also been influenced by the dietary practices of the Mediterranean countries, especially Greece. It's been demonstrated that olive oil, red wine, fish, and vegetables, which are abundant in the Mediterranean diet, are anticarcinogenic and contribute to the long lives of the people of this region. Even though the Mediterranean diet is high in fat (some studies have shown that almost 40 percent of its calories come from fat), it contains mostly monounsaturated and polyunsaturated fats—the kinds that are good for your health. Greeks are generally lean and have one of the lowest levels of heart disease in the world. Compare this with the American diet, which is almost 38 percent fat—most of it saturated fats, which contribute substantially to the prevalence of cardiovascular disease in the United States.

In fact, a study published in the *British Medical Journal* in 2005 looked at 74,000 healthy men and women over the age of sixty in nine European countries, and concluded that people in Greece and Spain (where they most closely follow a Mediterranean diet) had a significantly longer life expectancy than people in other countries.

WHEN IN PARIS . . .

I have no problem with "eating healthy" when I'm abroad. In fact, I usually lose weight without even trying. I eat normally; I drink the wine. I have a good time. I think our American food is so poisoned with chemicals and preservatives that it's really hard to eat a clean diet here. But in Europe, it's not laden with chemicals and preservatives, so I find it easier to eat healthier when I travel.

I'm a fish and vegetable person anyway. I eat that wherever I go, whether I'm here or I'm traveling. I'm pretty disciplined about my diet. I never eat on an airplane. I never drink alcohol on an airplane; I drink a lot of water. If you really have to have something, buy it before you fly and bring it with you.

If I were going out to dinner in Paris, a typical meal would be a salad and some fresh fish, a salmon or a turbot. The turbot is delicious there. The smoked salmon in Paris is different; it's not as salty. I don't know what they do to it, but all I can say is I eat a lot of it. When I do, my skin is clear; the bags under my eyes go away. I feel better; I look better. We're more challenged here to try to eat healthily just because of the way our food is prepared.

Also, I think the culture in Europe is that you don't eat between meals, and that you take your time to sit down for lunch and eat. When I'm in Paris, I follow the European tradition, which I don't do here. Here, I'm eating on the go, grabbing this, grabbing that. In France, I do as the Parisians do. I get up in the morning and I have a petit dejeuner (first meal of the day, roll and coffee or tea). Then I'm up and I'm out. Usually I have a lunch meeting, and I'll have a small salad or smoked salmon or something light. Maybe I'll stop and meet somebody for tea in the afternoon. At dinner, I'll have salad and fish and red wine. The portions are smaller than they serve here. At the end of the meal, maybe I'll try a little cheese or have a little dessert for a special occasion.

The way Europeans approach food, every meal is a celebration.

At lunch, you relax and you talk, even in the middle of the work day. Busy executives go to lunch. It's part of the lifestyle. And then you're not apt to reach for something unhealthy in the middle of the day. I think it's about structure and discipline. It takes time, and it takes thought, but it's doable. It's a different approach to life. It's a different quality of life that's lost here.

A meal in Europe is really about the experience. The focus on the family, getting together with the grandparents and aunts and uncles and cousins. The definition of family has changed so much in the United States. In Europe, it's a much closer unit. In their culture, it's all about la famille.

SUSAN TABAK, AGE FIFTY-ONE, FOUNDER OF
PARIS PERSONAL SHOPPER AND AUTHOR OF *CHIC IN PARIS*.

Defining the Mediterranean Diet

When people refer to the Mediterranean diet, they're actually referring to the traditional diet of the island of Crete prior to 1960. According to a 2001 article by Artemis P. Simopoulos in the *Journal of Nutrition*, presented at the 11th Annual Research Conference on Diet, Nutrition and Cancer (which was sponsored by the American Institute for Cancer Research), the Mediterranean diet resembles the Paleotech diet in amounts of fiber, antioxidants, saturated fat, monounsaturated fat, and the ratio of omega-6 to omega-3 fatty acids (a ratio of 2 to 1, as opposed to the current American ration of 16.74 to 1). The diet consists of foods rich in omega-3s (salmon, tuna, herring, mackerel, flaxseeds, green leafy vegetables), monounsaturated oils (olive and canola), seven or more servings of fruits and vegetables a day, lean meat, and low-fat dairy products. Simopoulos concluded that the traditional Greek diet, balanced in omega-6 and omega-3 fatty acids and rich in vitamins C and E from fruits and vegetables, "is associated with decreased rates of heart disease and cancer more so than any other diet or drug intervention."

Nutrition and Aging

There is one nutritional fact that we, with our Western sensibility, may find hard to swallow: We simply can't eat as much as we used to. When we were kids, we could eat all the time and burn it off easily. In our teens and twenties, when we were active all day and half the night, our energy output was at an all-time high. As we age, however, our metabolism naturally slows down. We have more body fat and less lean muscle. Therefore, we need to consume fewer calories (while following a program of muscle-building exercises, which is discussed in chapter 5). In addition, we must pay more attention to the quality of the foods we consume. A young body can process almost any kind of food, but as we get older our nutrient needs increase while our calorie needs decrease.

Getting the highest nutrient value from the food we eat is important throughout our lives, but it becomes even more important as we age. Eating right can help stave off the diseases prevalent among older people and can help improve the quality of life for those who already have some of these conditions. Many years of research and experience have taught me to appreciate the functional aspects of food—its inherent potential to improve energy; help maintain lean muscle mass; shore up aging immune systems; protect against heart disease, diabetes, and cancer; and enhance the overall quality of life. Now that we are living longer lives, this is more important than ever. I look at my parents and their generation, and I see how their eating habits (traditional Cuban fare with an emphasis on meat, saturated fats, and fried foods) have had a negative impact on their senior years. They did not have the benefit of the science of nutrition we now have at our fingertips.

The good news is that our approach to food is slowly changing. Super health food markets have sprung up next to traditional supermarkets. Farmers' markets are more popular than ever. It's becoming easier to lead healthy lives while taking pleasure in food. The goal is to design a diet that is therapeutic—with properties that reverse aging and improve overall performance—and enjoyable at the same time.

Efficiency Foods: The New 50 Fusion Food Plan

People come to see me for various reasons. Many want to lose weight, but most want to find a healthier lifestyle. They often come reluctantly, thinking they'll have to give up everything they love. I can't tell you how often I hear clients say, "I don't know if I can do this." It's clear to me that they don't know what "this" is. They think I'm going to put them on a restrictive program, but this eating program is about exploring the dietary landscape. After studying the efficiency of food, along with the culinary cultures of both Japan and the Mediterranean, I have taken the best from both and designed what I call the New 50 Fusion Food Plan.

Many baby boomers in their forties and fifties are still trying to diet in the same way they did when they were younger, thinking of food only in these terms: *Does it make me fat or does it make me thin?* This approach to dieting clearly doesn't work for the ever-increasing percentage of the population now deemed to be overweight. I believe we should be asking different questions about the food we eat: *Can it give me the energy I need to get through my day? Will it improve my immune response? Can it boost my mood? Will it feed my mind as well as my body?*

Efficiency foods (also called functional foods) are high-quality foods that are low on the glycemic index and high on the oxygen radical absorbance capacity (ORAC) scale (see sidebar). They contain phytochemicals (chemical compounds occurring naturally in plants) that work at molecular levels to help increase the efficiency of the body and longevity nutrients that go beyond vitamins and minerals. They help regulate hormones, control levels of cholesterol and homocysteine (an amino acid that is produced during metabolism and is believed to damage the lining cells of the arteries), and protect against osteoporosis. They aid in processing energy, improve the immune system, boost cognitive powers, and improve the health of skin and hair.

THE HIGHS AND LOWS OF EFFICIENCY FOODS

When you choose foods for their efficiency values, there are two indicators that can help you decide. One is the glycemic index, which measures how rapidly a carbohydrate is absorbed into your bloodstream and its potential impact on insulin secretion. The higher a food's glycemic value, the faster it enters the bloodstream. When that happens, the pancreas responds by secreting insulin. That brings your blood sugar levels down, but it also signals the body to store fat.

The second efficiency value can be found on the ORAC scale, which measures the total antioxidant power of foods. Studies done at the U.S. Department of Agriculture's (USDA's) Human Nutrition Research Center on Aging at Tufts University suggest that eating plenty of high-ORAC fruits and vegetables may help "slow the processes associated with aging in both body and brain." High-ORAC foods include fruits such as prunes, blackberries, blueberries, and strawberries and vegetables such as kale, spinach, Brussels sprouts, and broccoli.

You can find lists of both glycemic values and ORAC values of foods on dozens of sites on the Internet, including www.glycemicindex.com, www. diabetesnet.com, and www.ars.usda.gov//SP2Userfiles/place/12354500/Data/ ORAC/ORAC07.pdf.

The following list of efficiency foods is not all-inclusive, but it contains what I consider to be the must-haves for a healthy diet.

ESSENTIAL EFFICIENCY FOODS

VEGETABLES

Artichokes

Alfalfa sprouts

Arugula

Asparagus

Bean sprouts

Bok choy

Broccoli

Broccoli sprouts

Brussels sprouts

Cabbage

Cauliflower

Carrots

Celery

Cucumbers

Endives

Garlic

Green beans

Kale

Leeks

Lettuce

Mixed field greens

Mushrooms

Onions

Parsley

Peppers

Radishes

Scallions

Shallots

Spinach

Squash

Tomatoes

Turnips

Watercress

Zucchini

FRUITS

Apples

Açai

Avocados

Blackberries

Blueberries

Cherries

Figs

Goji berries

Lemons

Mangoes

Melons

Oranges

Papayas

Pomegranates

Raspberries

Red grapefruits

Strawberries

SEAFOOD

Anchovies

Codfish

12

Bass
Flounder
Haddock
Halibut
Herring
Mackerel
Mahi-mahi
Monkfish
Salmon
Sardines
Scallops
Shrimp
Snapper
Sole
Tuna
Turbot
Seaweed

LEAN POULTRY
Chicken
Duck
Eggs (egg whites or Egg
  Beaters)
Guinea hens
Turkey

BEANS AND LEGUMES
Adzuki beans
Black beans
Chickpeas
Lentils
Soybeans

WHOLE GRAINS
Buckwheat
Corn
Integral rice (*e.g.*, whole rice, brown
  rice, basmati rice)
Millet
Oatmeal
Quinoa
Rye
Spelt
Wheat germ

STARCHES
Pumpkin
Sweet potatoes
Squash (*e.g.,* acorn, butternut,
  spaghetti, yellow,
  zucchini)
Yams

NUTS AND SEEDS
Almonds
Brazil nuts
Cashews
Flaxseeds
Macadamia nuts
Pecans
Walnuts

DAIRY
Bio-yogurt (see box on Probiotics on
  page 23)

13

Cottage cheese

Feta cheese

Goat cheese

Mozzarella

Parmigiano reggiano

Sheep cheese

Yogurt

SPICES, HERBS, AND
CONDIMENTS

Anise

Basil

Cardamom

Cayenne pepper

Chili powder

Chives

Cilantro

Cinnamon

Chili pepper

Coriander

Cumin

Curry powder

Fenugreek

Ginger

Himalayan crystal salt

Hummus

Mint

Nutmeg

Oregano

Paprika

Rosemary

Saffron

Sage

Salsa

Sea salt

Tarragon

Thyme

Turmeric

Wasabi

ADDITIONAL EFFICIENCY
FOODS

Artisanal honey

Canola oil

Chocolate (70 percent to 80 percent
  dark)

Extra-virgin olive oil

Grapeseed oil

Tea (white, green, oolong,
  black)

Stevia

Whey shakes

Making Healthy Choices

Again, the list above is just to give you an idea of the kinds of foods that contribute to healthy aging. When you're making dietary choices, here are some other factors to consider:

CARBOHYDRATES: Carbohydrates have gotten a bad rap lately—in part, deservedly so. Carbs found in foods such as bread, pasta, cakes, cookies, pizza, fast foods, ice cream, candy, and anything with refined sugar cause the tissues in our bodies to become rigid and pigmented (producing age spots) and to form advanced glycation end products (AGEs), which accumulate in our bodies as we get older. These AGEs glue themselves to collagen, veins, arteries, ligaments, bones, brains—just about everywhere in the body—and cause stiff joints, hardened arteries, weakened muscles, and organ deterioration. Clearly, the further you stay away from these kinds of carbs, the better. However, not all carbohydrates are bad. Paleocarbs, another category of carbohydrates associated with the Paleotech diet, are low in glycemic impact and high in the kind of phytochemicals that fight free radicals (molecular terrorists that attack cells in the body). Paleocarbs are found in legumes, beans and bean products, root vegetables such as yams and squash, and grains such as quinoa, millet, oats, and brown rice.

A Word about Wheat and Whole Grains: I refer to wheat as a "dietary sponge." It causes most people to gain weight, have increased appetites, retain fluids, and escalate inflammation. Wheat contains both lectins, proteins that bind to sugars or other carbohydrates, and gluten, a portion of the grain that is difficult for most people to assimilate and that has been linked to many physical disorders—from arthritis to schizophrenia to a host of digestive diseases. I recommend that you stay away from wheat as much as possible, and look instead for whole grains like barley, brown rice, and oatmeal. Whole grains consist of three components: the bran, the germ, and the endosperm. Refined grains have been stripped of the bran and the germ, which means they have lost most of their B vitamins, minerals, and fiber. When you eat grains without their fiber, the carbohydrates quickly turn to glucose and enter the bloodstream. Carbohydrates in whole grains, which have their fiber intact, are not absorbed as quickly. This regulates blood sugar and also keeps you from getting hungry again for a while. If you're trying to bulk up

15

TWO GREAT WAYS TO BE FRUITFUL

It's easy to get overwhelmed with all the choices of foods out there. We often get into a rut of eating only those foods that are familiar to us. That doesn't mean you need to give up the tried and true just for the sake of variety. I usually suggest that people try something new every once in a while as an adjunct to their old favorites. Two fruits, one that everyone knows and loves, and one that may not be part of your normal shopping list, have been shown to be particularly beneficial: blueberries and pomegranates.

- When the U.S. Department of Agriculture tested more than one hundred different fruits, vegetables, nuts, herbs, and spices for total antioxidant capacity per serving, one food came out on top: blueberries. Among the many benefits of this tiny fruit are maintaining arterial structure and regulating blood pressure, improving memory, reversing brain aging, protecting against brain ischemia (interruption of blood flow to the brain), and inhibiting metastasis (stopping cancerous cells from invading surrounding tissue). In fact, there is strong evidence to show that blueberries protect against most age-related illnesses.

- The pomegranate, which has long been known as the jewel of winter, has recently become known for its high antioxidant content. Pomegranate juice is high in three different types of polyphenols—tannins, anthocyanins, and ellagic acid—that are potent forms of antioxidants. Studies have shown that pomegranate juice contains three times the total antioxidant ability of green tea or red wine, and is high in potassium, fiber, vitamin C, and niacin. And, in February 2006, *Men's Health* magazine reported on a study by the Preventive Medicine Research Institute in Sausalito, California, which suggested that pomegranate juice might help stave off heart attacks. Scientists gave eight ounces of juice daily to a group of patients who had experienced poor blood circulation to their hearts, a strong indicator of future heart attacks. After three months, their blood flow had improved by an average of 17 percent, which researchers attributed to the pomegranate's high levels of artery-clearing antioxidants.

your fiber intake, look for whole grains. According to the National Academy of Sciences, men over the age of fifty should consume at least thirty grams a day, and women in the same age group should consume at least twenty-one grams. (Most Americans currently consume only between five and thirteen grams.)

PROTEINS: Although I usually advocate what I call a Paleotech diet—sticking as closely as possible to what our early ancestors ate—that's not always possible in the modern world. Prehistoric people ate a high-protein diet, but the animal protein they consumed was not like the kind we find in today's supermarkets. The proteins they ate contained no synthetic hormones or preservatives. The animals they consumed were lean and muscular, full of unsaturated fats like omega-3 fatty acids. The meat we eat today, especially beef, comes from grain-fed animals full of saturated fat.

One thing you can do to counteract this tendency is to choose organic meats whenever possible. Organic meats are free of synthetic pesticides and chemicals, artificial additives, and preservatives. They are given organic feed that contains no growth hormones and are reared without the routine use of antibiotics.

A Word about Soy: Soy is a protein source very rich in chemicals called isoflavones, plant substances that closely resemble the female hormone estrogen. That's why many women who are perimenopausal and menopausal do well with soy products added to their diets. I recommend

17

using soy the way the Japanese do—in small amounts of whole soy foods such as tofu and edamame, and in fermented versions such as miso soup and tempeh. Avoid commercialized soy products such as soy hot dogs, ice cream, and cookies, which are high in isoflavones but are lacking in protein, calcium, and essential fatty acids.

FATS: Because the word "fat" has so many negative connotations in our society, many people believe they have to cut fat completely out of their diets. This is an unhealthy mistake, made by most people concerned about their weight and their cholesterol levels. The unfortunate result has been a great reduction in the consumption of omega-3 fatty acids. Omega-3 fatty acids are considered essential fatty acids, which means that they are essential to human health but cannot be manufactured by the body and must be obtained from food. Omega-3 (and omega-6, another essential fatty acid) plays a crucial role in brain function as well as in normal growth and development. These essential fatty acids are highly concentrated in the brain and appear to be particularly important for cognitive and behavioral function. Research has shown that omega-3 fatty acids decrease the risk of arrhythmias, which can lead to sudden cardiac death; they also decrease triglyceride levels, decrease the growth rate of plaque in the arteries, and can help lower blood pressure.

The American Heart Association's dietary guidelines recommend that healthy adults eat at least two servings of fish per week, particularly fish such as mackerel, lake trout, herring, sardines, albacore tuna, and salmon. These fish contain two omega-3 fatty acids: eicosapentaenoic acid (EPA) and docosa-hexaenoic acid (DHA).

A Word about Olive Oil: The ancient Greek physician Hippocrates (460–370 BC), known as the father of medicine, was the first to mention the health benefits of olive oil. Many recent studies have supported his findings. In the September 2005 issue of *Nature* magazine, a report by Paul A. S. Breslin of the Monell Chemical Senses Center in Philadelphia stated that he and his fellow researchers had discovered an important reason for the positive effect of olive oil on cardiovascular health: it contains oleocanthal, a substance that has the same anti-inflammatory effects as drugs like ibuprofen and aspirin. The study found that extra-virgin olive oil is the most beneficial. Dr. Breslin suggested that the Mediterranean diet, which makes liberal use of extra-virgin olive oil on bread, vegetables, and in salad dressing, may be the best way to consume it. Another article, titled "The Effect of Polyphenols in Olive Oil on Heart Disease Risk Factors" by María-Isabel Covas, MS, PhD, et al., published in the September 5, 2006, issue of the *Annals of Internal Medicine*, reported that virgin olive oil (oil that comes from the first pressing of the olives and has no more than 2 percent oleic acid, a monounsaturated fat) contains a high level of antioxidant plant compounds called polyphenols, which have been shown to be particularly effective at lowering the risk of heart disease.

Tips for Following the New 50 Fusion Food Plan

19

- Eat several small meals throughout the day, as opposed to three large ones.
- Start your day with a good breakfast within an hour of waking, even if you don't feel like eating. It's the best way to rev up your energy and get your brain properly fueled for the day.
- Have a mini-meal or snack between breakfast and lunch.
- Have a light dinner, and if you're hungry later in the evening, have a light snack (for instance, a small amount of fruit or even a bit of high-quality semisweet chocolate).
- Structure your meals around a primary protein, either seafood or dairy. Add a vegetable component and a starch component.
- Go for variety. You don't need to have lots of different foods within a single day, but mix things up during the week. Variety will keep you entertained and will allow you to enjoy your meals more fully.

A Day in the Life of the New 50 Fusion Food Plan

I can't be on a diet where everything is flavorless—fish with nothing on it, plain steamed veggies, salad with only lemon juice. That's not how I want to live. In order to show how this works in the real world (or *my* real world, anyway), I've outlined below what I typically eat in a twenty-four-hour period. I've given several suggestions for each meal or snack. You don't have to eat exactly what I eat, but I've found that this program of healthy eating works for me and most of my clients.

BREAKFAST: This meal is the most different from what Americans traditionally eat in the morning. It may take some getting used to, but these choices give me a healthy start for the day.

- *Breakfast Shakes*: I often start the day with a shake made with Designer Protein powder (a whey protein product that is pure, natural, high-quality protein from cow's milk and a rich source of essential amino acids. It's almost 100 percent lactose free for the lactose intolerant). I pour two scoops of Designer Protein in a blender, add twelve ounces of water, one teaspoon of yogurt, and a small handful of frozen berries, papaya, or mango, then blend, pour, and drink. Another option is an UltraClear shake (made from rice-protein concentrate and designed to be used as part of a detoxification program—which is discussed further in the next chapter).
- *Japanese Style*: I'll have a small amount of cooked brown basmati rice; about four ounces of either salmon, salmon salad, tuna, or tuna salad; and a small assortment of vegetables that have been steamed or stir-fried the night before, or a small salad. Sometimes I start the day with a small portion of miso soup.
- *Hearty Meal*: On a cold winter day, I often have a bowl of bean soup. Two of my favorites are Coco Pazzo Five Bean and Health Valley

Black Bean (I sometimes add a drizzle of olive oil to give it a little kick). Another hearty choice is a bowl of oatmeal with some stevia (a noncaloric natural sugar substitute) and cinnamon for flavor. If I want something starchy, I'll have 100 percent flaxseed bread or sunflower-seed bread.

- *Organic Eggs*: Breakfast can also be two poached organic eggs with a slice of flaxseed, sunflower-seed, or 100 percent rye-flour bread (avoid anything that's wheat based). Some mornings I'll have a hard-boiled egg, a can of sardines, and a slice of rye or flax bread.

- *Cereal*: I don't often have cereal for breakfast (only because I personally prefer the other options listed here), but if I do, I usually choose Kashi Go Lean and have it with rice milk or soy milk. I'll sweeten it with honey or stevia and add blueberries and/or strawberries for their rich antioxidant properties. I might also accompany this meal with a glass of pomegranate juice.

LUNCH: Lunch is not usually a major meal, but it is another opportunity to add fuel in the form of protein to keep me going for the rest of the day.

- *Salad Nicoise*: This is usually a homemade version consisting of a bed of greens with seared tuna or seared salmon. I may add a hard-boiled egg and a few olives, drizzled with olive oil and balsamic vinegar.

- *Broiled Fish*: I often pair a broiled salmon steak with steamed or stir-fried vegetables, especially spinach, which is high in lutein and zeaxanthin, antioxidants that protect against macular degeneration (the leading cause of legal blindness in Americans over age fifty-five). I may also have a few slices of tomato for the antioxidant lycopene, which is found in red vegetables and fruits and known to be effective against cancer—particularly prostate cancer.

- *Avocado Salad*: I love having a plate of freshly sliced avocado and tomato, and feta or mozzarella cheese, drizzled with extra-virgin olive oil.

DINNER: Dinner is sometimes the largest meal of the day if I'm going out with friends, but I try to keep it small as often as possible. This is not difficult if I've had small snacks throughout the day.

- *Broiled Fish*: This could be tuna, salmon, or halibut, or for a change, a shrimp-based dish. I like to garnish this dish with salads, and steamed or stir-fried vegetables including broccoli, cabbage, kale, cauliflower, or Brussels sprouts. All of these foods contain the cancer-fighting antioxidant indole 3 carbonyls and are also a good source of fiber. If I want a starch, I'll add quinoa, whole-grain basmati rice, or a starchy vegetable like squash, yam, or sweet potato. Typically, I garnish these with olive oil and spices.
- *Other Options*: On very rare occasions, I will eat red meat (preferably organic). I occasionally eat lamb, chicken, or turkey, but I tend to choose fish most often.

SNACKS: I try to have at least two snacks a day, between breakfast and lunch, and lunch and dinner. I sometimes have an after-dinner snack as well.

- *Yogurt and Fruit*: I choose good-quality yogurt that contains probiotics (see sidebar), and add sliced papaya or mango, or fruit salad that contains cantaloupe, grapes, and berries.
- *Feta Cheese*: I enjoy feta cheese on a slice of rye bread or a rye cracker.
- *Fresh Turkey*: I'll pair this with a few slices of tomato drizzled with olive oil.
- *Canned Fish*: I might just open a can of sardines or tuna packed in water and eat as is.
- *Power Bar*: Power bars can be great if you're in a hurry and need a quick energy boost. But be sure to read the label—not all power bars are the same. You want the ones with the lowest amount of fat and sugar (ten grams or less), and the highest amount of protein (twenty grams or more).

PROBIOTICS

The word "probiotic" means, literally, "for life." Probiotics are beneficial bacteria that can actually help strengthen the body's natural defenses and restore the appropriate balance of healthy bacteria. Unlike antibiotics, which are used to kill off harmful bacteria, probiotics are used to boost the amount of protective bacteria in our systems. The balance of harmful versus protective bacteria can be thrown off by a wide range of circumstances including the overuse of antibiotics or other drugs (legal and otherwise), excess alcohol, stress, disease, and exposure to toxic substances. Certain foods contain probiotics in therapeutic amounts, such as yogurt that is labeled to have "live cultures." The beneficial properties of dairy foods containing live cultures have been recognized for hundreds of years; they promote good digestion, boost immune function, and help prevent vaginal yeast infections.

- *Nuts*: A handful of almonds, cashews, walnuts, or Brazil nuts can be good for you because they are rich sources of omega-3 fatty acids.

As I said before, I don't expect you to eat what I eat. I eat what I like and what works for me. The great thing about the New 50 Fusion Food Plan is that it is so flexible. Choose foods that suit your personal taste and fit within your nutritional needs (taking into account any allergies you may have, or restrictions based on illness or health issues). Keep the list of efficiency foods on page 12 handy and include as many of them as possible in your daily diet. You don't have to be perfect at every meal—that's not what life is about. But if you increase the number of healthy choices you make each day, you increase the potential of extending the health of your life.

MIXING IT UP

To me, eating well means leading a healthy lifestyle. Not going on crazy diets. I never went on weeks of fasting or not eating. I went through the obligatory phase in my twenties of trying to be a vegetarian, but as I've gotten older, I find it's all about a balance of eating properly and exercising every day and not being a fanatic about anything.

Except I think you should be fanatic about one thing: whatever you put into your mouth, ask yourself, "How does this benefit me?" That makes it difficult to eat without thinking. If you cook that way and you eat that way, it's really just as easy as eating things that aren't good for you.

There's no typical meal I might have; it changes from day to day. I like to cook, so that makes it easy. I do not make food a religion—I wouldn't say I have to eat red meat every day or I'm a vegetarian every day. The best thing is to mix it up. I make a concoction in the morning with a lot of things that Oz recommends: a shake in the morning, fresh fruit. Then I'll have an egg and maybe some spinach. If I'm having a hard-boiled egg, at the last minute I'll throw in a bunch of spinach or kale, then drain it, and have it with some flax bread. I never get to the point where I'm starving, I'm always eating something, whether it's yogurt with some nuts thrown in, or a sandwich filled with leftover vegetables from the night before. If you have just vegetables, you're going to be starving an hour later, especially if you're active. So I'll have some great bread with it.

If I'm making soup, even if it's traditional chicken soup, at the very end I'll throw in a ton of fresh greens so that they're cooking for just for a few minutes and stay bright green and crunchy. I have red meat every once in a while. If I'm craving something sweet for dessert, I get raw organic chocolate, grind it up, and sprinkle it over fruit. It's delicious. Or I'll make a shake with frozen bananas in the middle of the day if I'm hungry, and I'll put in a little bit of honey and fresh vanilla and maybe that little square of the dark chocolate. If you can't have milk, you can make it with rice milk. It tastes great. Just because it's healthy, it doesn't have to be bland and boring.

RICKI LUBART, FIFTY-ONE,
MARRIED, MOTHER

CLEANING HOUSE

DETOXING FOR HEALTH

THERE IS NO better way to embark on the *Redesigning 50* program than by "cleaning house" with a powerful detoxification regimen. Detoxification is the process by which toxins—poisonous compounds in the body—are eliminated from the body or are changed into less toxic substances. Toxins are everywhere in the modern world. They're in the food we eat, the water we drink, even the air we breathe. If you're alive, you're ingesting or inhaling one toxic substance or another all day, every day. It only makes sense, then, to clean the body out on a regular basis.

Toxins tend to concentrate in the liver and the gastrointestinal tract. If you are in perfect health, these organs will eliminate much of the "junk" that accumulates in the body. However, the unending exposure to toxins in our world makes it difficult for the body to keep up and keep clean. Toxins build up, drain our energy, and make us more susceptible to disease and infection.

I learned this early in my life when I first began exploring nutrition. I suffered from terrible migraine headaches and searched for years for some relief, but I didn't find it until I learned the basics of detoxification. I began slowly by reducing or eliminating my intake of certain foods, some of which I'd eaten all my life. I gave up sugar, fried foods, coffee, and smoking. I greatly reduced the amount of red meat in my diet. I went on juice fasts and started meditation. As a result, I had fewer and fewer headaches.

The science of detoxification has advanced a great deal since then. There are several ways to aid your body's natural detoxing processes. Here are some of them:

- Include protein at every meal (protein is rich in the detoxifying enzyme glutathione).
- Drink six to eight glasses of water a day to flush out impurities.
- Feast on fiber (especially cruciferous vegetables such as broccoli, kale, cauliflower, and cabbage, as well as fruits such as apples and berries).
- Include antioxidants from red, green, and yellow vegetables, raw seeds, and nuts.
- Increase omega-3 fatty acids.
- Avoid refined carbohydrates, which slow down the activity of detoxifying enzymes.

If you really want to do a thorough cleansing, however, you can embark on a full-blown weeklong detox program. Starting a health management program with a thorough detoxification can be extremely beneficial. (*Caution:* a detox program like the following one should be done only with proper guidance, especially if it's your first time.)

I'd heard about Adina Niemerow through friends. She is a holistic chef who has studied with Paul Pitchford (author of *Healing with Whole Foods*) and at the Natural Gourmet holistic culinary school. She's worked with many celebrities, including Steve Jobs of Apple Computers and designer Donna Karan. She's an expert on detoxification and the author of *SuperCleanse: 10 Rejuvenating Detox Treatments for Body, Beauty, and Spirit.* We invited her to describe a typical cleanse she would design if she were to be someone's "personal food trainer" for a week.

Notes from Adina

For the past twelve years, unlocking the transformative power of whole foods to cleanse and rejuvenate the body, mind, and spirit has been my passion. On this journey, I've been fortunate to work and study with some of the foremost health professionals and chefs in the "healing foods" arena, including Paul Pitchford, author of *Healing with Whole Foods*, Dr. Gabriel Cousens, founder of the Tree of Life center in Arizona, and Dr. David Jubb of Jubb's Longevity Center in New York.

Over the years, I've incorporated the lessons I've learned into a cleanse program that has helped hundreds of my clients reset their bodies and lives—whether they've been battling disease, depression, or addiction; striving to lose weight; or simply seeking greater levels of energy and focus. I am always thrilled to work with clients and help them experience firsthand the dramatic and positive changes that a cleanse can accomplish in our lives.

I start by putting a client on a clean diet—that is, a diet of foods free of all substances that wreak havoc on our bodies, including chemicals, additives, hormones, caffeine, and anything containing refined white flour or sugar. The impact of a clean diet is amazing—especially for people in their fifties—not only in the way they feel but also in the way they look. It boosts energy, increases flexibility, and dramatically improves the health and appearance of eyes, skin, and hair.

The seven-day regimen I designed for this book is predominantly a green juice cleanse, low in natural sugars. Greens emulsify cholesterol and fat in the body and detoxify the liver. And if you live in a city, they boost the amount of chlorophyll in the body, which city dwellers really need. The green juices I created include combinations of kale, spinach, parsley, cucumber, celery, fennel, apple, ginger, carrot, rainbow chard, dandelion, lemon, and turmeric.

As toxins are flushed from the body you may experience a spectrum of aches and emotions, so here are some helpful tips you can use to maximize the cleanse and ease the process:

- Take Epsom salt or aromatherapy baths before bed to relax, reduce body aches, and pull toxins from the body.

- Make an appointment for a massage or energy work. I recommend at least one lymphatic massage. Working with a skilled healer during the cleanse makes profound, positive shifts in your life force energy.
- Drink plenty of water. You can add Himalayan crystal salt for extra minerals and flavor (or drink Oz Water, which already contains Himalayan crystal salt and can be ordered online at www.ozgarcia .com). You can drink any high-quality bottled water. My favorites are Fiji, Vitamin Water, and Oz Water. You can also use a home water purifier such as Brita or Pur, if you prefer.
- To ensure that you continue to be regular (there is no fiber in the cleanse juices), take one teaspoon in the morning and one teaspoon in the evening of Ionic Fizz Powder by Pure Essence or Mag-Tea G Powder by Douglas Laboratories.
- Sweat the toxins out of your body by using a sauna or steam.
- Do only light exercise such as stretching, yoga, or easy walks.
- Keep a journal. During a fast, the mind becomes clearer, and many people experience real breakthroughs and find clarity on issues that have been weighing them down. This is a great time to set intentions for the months ahead and to take time out to look at how you're taking care of yourself.

The Seven-Day Cleanse Program

For the duration of the cleanse, you should refrain from all alcohol, caffeine, red meat, white flour products (such as pasta and bread), hydrogenated fats, preservatives, refined sugar, dairy, and fried foods. You start the first day with four green juices every three hours.

If the juices alone prove to be too extreme for the middle of a hectic week and you want something more substantial to sustain you during the day, you can add a mineral broth made of sweet potatoes, shiitake mushrooms, burdock, leeks, celery, parsley, ginger, kombu seaweed, marine minerals, Himalayan crystal salt, and ground flaxseeds. The broth will satisfy your appetite and make the cleanse easier.

Day One

- Start the day by drinking one to two cups of hot water with a squeeze of lemon.
- Drink four to five 16-ounce glasses of green juices daily. Drinking the juice every three hours works to keep energy flowing. I suggest the following schedule: 8:00 a.m., 11:00 a.m., 2:00 p.m., 5:00 p.m., and 8:00 p.m.
- Drink water throughout the day, including water mixed with lemon and a pinch of Himalayan crystal salt and MSM (methylsulfonylmethane, an organic sulfur compound that appears in all living organisms). MSM is great for maintaining skin elasticity, protecting connective tissue and joint cartilage, reducing scar tissue and inflammation, and relieving arthritic conditions. It is sold in powdered form at many health food stores. Young coconut water is also allowed because of its high concentration of electrolytes (it can be very sweet, so water it down).
- Drink tea throughout the day. You may include tea that has licorice, black sesame seeds, anise flower, peppermint, ginger, chrysanthemum flowers, chamomile, fennel, and tulsi (an Indian herb rich in antioxidants). Most blends of caffeine-free, stimulant-free, and bedtime calming teas found at local health food stores include some combination of these ingredients.

Day Two

- Start the day by drinking hot water with a squeeze of lemon.
- Drink three 16-ounce glasses of green juices throughout the day: one at 8:00 a.m., one at 11:00 a.m., and one at 2:00 p.m. These juices are available at many health food stores or specialty markets, or you can make them at home if you have a juicer (recipes are included in the next section).

- Enjoy two 16-ounce bowls of mineral broth during the rest of the afternoon and early evening (see the recipe for mineral broth in the next section).
- Continue drinking lots of tea and water.
- Get a massage or energy work.
- Go for a light walk.
- Take a hot bath.

Day Three

- Follow the same juice and broth schedule as on Day Two.
- Drink plenty of water and teas.
- Take a hot bath.

Day Four

- Follow the same schedule of juice and broth.
- Get a massage.
- Go for a light walk.
- Take a hot/cold plunge. Plunges, also known as hydrotherapy, have recuperative healing properties. Generally, heat has a calming effect and slows down the activity of internal organs, while cold acts as a stimulant and speeds up internal activity.
- Get a five- to ten-minute steam or sauna at a local spa or gym to sweat out toxins and purify the body. Infrared saunas are especially good, if there's one nearby.

Day Five

- Follow the same juice and broth schedule.
- Go for a light walk.

- Get energy work or a shiatsu massage to move energy through the body.
- Dry-brush the body to invigorate the skin. Use a soft-bristle brush, and brush the limbs and belly in the direction of the heart. This helps eliminate toxins and stimulate the lymphatic system.
- Take a hot bath.
- Go to bed early.

Day Six

- Follow the same juice and broth schedule.
- Drink plenty of water and teas.
- Take a vitamin and mineral supplement.
- Go for a light walk.
- Get a massage and facial.
- Take a hot bath.

31

Day Seven

- Follow the same juice and broth schedule.
- Take a steam or sauna, or get a massage.
- Take a hot bath near bedtime.

Breaking the Cleanse

Once you complete the cleanse, it's time to introduce yourself to a new way of eating. Breaking the fast with enzyme-rich foods is crucial. Once our bodies are cleansed of toxins, we respond quickly to healthy, life-force food—we may even get a "high" from eating the right foods. I suggest you start with live foods (foods that haven't been cooked), and add probiotics (available at your local health food store) to rebuild the digestive system.

It is best to begin with live foods because heat destroys the natural enzymes in foods and makes them harder to digest. Poorly digested food isn't easily eliminated from the body and tends to leave behind particles that turn into acidic waste. Conversely, the natural enzymes in live foods aid the digestive process, moving food through the body and freeing up the energy the body expends by trying to break down food for other purposes.

On the first day after your fast, I would introduce fruits and salads to your diet. Then we would move on to nutrient-rich salad dressings, enzyme-packed smoothies and soups, and slowly start a well-balanced, low-glycemic diet.

Recipes for Breaking the Cleanse

I use the following recipes, which I've created and collected over several years while working with Dr. David Jubb of Jubb's Longevity Center in New York and Dr. Gabriel Cousens's Tree of Life Cafe in Patagonia, Arizona. Be sure to wash all vegetables and fruit thoroughly before using, and use organic produce whenever possible.

ALIVE CARROT SOUP

*Makes 4 cups (either 4 appetizer servings or
2 main course servings)*

4 cups organic carrot juice (you can buy this at a juice bar or health food
    store, or make it yourself with about 4 large carrots, if you have a
    juicer)
4 medium carrots
½ ripe avocado, peeled and pitted

1 tablespoon fresh ginger root, peeled and minced

1 teaspoon fresh mint, chopped

1 teaspoon fresh basil, chopped

1 jalapeño pepper, seeded and chopped (more or less to taste, but
beware—a little goes a long way!)

Pinch of Himalayan crystal salt (can be purchased at many health food
stores or online; you can also substitute any high-quality salt)

1 teaspoon fresh-squeezed lime juice (or more to taste)

OPTIONAL GARNISHES

1 cup sprouts (I use sunflower sprouts, but any sprouts will do)

½ cucumber, peeled and chopped

1 tablespoon fresh cilantro, chopped

½ ripe avocado, chopped into small pieces

Pinch of cayenne pepper

1. Pour the carrot juice into a blender.
2. Add the avocado, ginger, mint, basil, jalapeno, salt, and lime juice. Blend until smooth.
3. Add more lime juice and salt to taste.
4. Serve in bowls. Arrange an attractive pattern of garnishes atop each bowl of soup just before serving. You can use small pieces of many different herbs, sprouts, and vegetables for garnish. Choose a few that you like, and sprinkle on top of the soup.

MINERAL BROTH

Makes 8 cups

Make your mineral broth the night before you start your cleanse. It will last up to three days in the refrigerator.

2 cups celery (about 3 to 4 stalks, chopped)

2 cups yellow onion (about 2 medium onions, chopped)

2 cups leeks (about 1 large or 2 medium leeks, chopped)

1 cup fresh burdock root, chopped (a 6- to 9-inch piece of burdock root)

1 cup fresh shiitake mushrooms, or 1 cup dried 4-inch piece of kombu
(a sea vegetable found at local health food stores or Asian markets)

4 tablespoons ginger, chopped

2 cups carrots (about 3 medium carrots, chopped)

10 cloves garlic (separated, but not peeled)

12 sprigs parsley

3 medium yams, halved (washed, but not peeled)

Himalayan sea salt to taste

Cayenne pepper to taste

1 teaspoon fresh ginger, minced (optional)

1. In a 5-quart stock pot, combine the celery, onions, leeks, burdock root, shiitake mushrooms or kombu, chopped ginger, carrots, garlic cloves, parsley, and yams, leaving the yams on top.

2. Fill the stock pot with cold water to 1 inch from the top.

3. Bring the water to a boil, then reduce the heat. Simmer the broth on the stove top for 1½ hours.

4. Turn heat off, and let broth cool for at least 30 minutes.

5. When broth is cool, strain the cooked vegetables into a colander. Pull out the yams and set them aside. Discard the rest of the vegetables.

6. In small batches, mix the liquid broth and pieces of unpeeled yams in a blender until you get a light soup consistency.

7. Add salt to taste (but go easy).

8. Add cayenne to taste (beware—a little goes a long way).

9. Add the optional teaspoon of minced fresh ginger if you'd like more heat and flavor.

GREEN DRINKS

Makes 3 cups (two 2-ounce servings)

1 cucumber, peeled and chopped

3 stalks celery, cut into 2-inch pieces

1 apple, cored and chopped

$\frac{1}{2}$ cup fennel (about 1 small fennel, chopped)

$\frac{1}{2}$ cup kale (about 2 leaves, chopped)

$\frac{1}{2}$ cup rainbow chard (about 2 leaves)

2 to 3 sprigs parsley, chopped

OPTIONAL GARNISH

1 slice or a squeeze of fresh lemon

1. Put the cucumber, celery, apple, and fennel into one bowl and the kale, chard, and parsley into another.
2. Run all the ingredients through the feed tube of a high-powered juicer, alternating between the greens and the hard vegetables. This will prevent the juicer from having any difficulty juicing the greens.
3. Serve immediately in a large glass with a slice or squeeze of lemon. If you're new to green juices, it may take you some time to appreciate the flavor. If that's the case, dilute the juice with some water, and squeeze in a bit more lemon to taste.

35

BROCCOLI HEMPSEED SALAD

Makes 2 servings

2 cups broccoli florets (about $\frac{1}{2}$-inch pieces, coarsely chopped)

Pinch of Himalayan sea salt

½ cup cherry tomatoes, halved

4 green olives, pitted and quartered

⅛ cup hempseeds (can be purchased at your local health food store or
  ordered online at www.rawfood.com; if you cannot locate them, you
  can substitute sesame seeds or flaxseeds)

2 tablespoons olive oil (preferably organic, cold pressed)

1 teaspoon lemon juice (or more, to taste)

1. In a salad bowl, mix the chopped broccoli florets and the sea salt together
   with your hands. Then massage, knead, and squeeze the broccoli with your
   hands until it begins to wilt a bit and feel damp on your hands. This breaks
   down the fibers, making it more digestible.

2. Add the tomatoes, olives, hempseeds, olive oil, and lemon juice. Toss and
   serve.

KALE AVOCADO SALAD

Makes 2 servings

5 or 6 large kale leaves

Pinch of Himalayan sea salt

1 avocado, peeled and pitted

Fresh-squeezed lime juice to taste

1 cup tomatoes, chopped

3 tablespoons fresh cilantro, chopped

¼ cup Eden Shake (a condiment available at Whole Foods Market; if
  not available, substitute an additional pinch or two of salt and
  2 tablespoons sesame seeds)

1. Wash, dry, and remove the stems from the kale. Then stack up the leaves and
   roll them up like a burrito. While holding the kale in a roll, slice it very thinly.

2. In a salad bowl, add the sea salt to the sliced kale. Mix it in with your hands and then massage, knead, and squeeze the kale with your hands until it begins to wilt a bit and feel damp on your hands. This breaks down the fibers, making it more digestible.

3. Add the avocado and the lime juice. Using your hands or a wooden spoon, mash them into the kale.

4. Toss in the tomatoes, the cilantro, and the Eden Shake.

5. Serve immediately, or let rest at room temperature for up to 15 to 20 minutes before serving. For best results, do not refrigerate. (This dish does take a bit of extra chewing, so don't try to eat it in a hurry!)

RED PEPPER PÂTÉ NORI ROLLS

Makes 4 entrée servings, or 8 appetizer servings

FOR THE RED PEPPER PÂTÉ

1 cup macadamia nuts

1 cup red peppers, roughly chopped

2 tablespoons lemon juice, fresh squeezed

3 tablespoons fresh cilantro, finely chopped

Pinch of Himalayan sea salt

3 tablespoons green olives, pitted and chopped

FOR THE NORI ROLLS

2 cups baby lettuce leaves or larger lettuce leaves, chopped into 2-inch pieces

½ cup carrots (about 1 carrot, thinly julienned)

½ cup cucumber (about ½ a cucumber, thinly julienned)

1 avocado, peeled, pitted, and thinly sliced

8 Nori seaweed sheets (available at specialty grocers, health food stores, and Asian markets)

½ teaspoon wasabi paste, also known as Japanese horseradish (optional)

1. For the red pepper pâté: In a food processor, blend all the pâté ingredients into a rough, chunky consistency. Remove from the food processor and put into a bowl for immediate use, or cover and refrigerate for up to two days before moving to the next step.

2. To assemble the Nori rolls, spread 2 to 3 spoonfuls of the red pepper pâté across one of the short ends of each Nori sheet, and top with a few pieces each of the lettuce, cucumbers, carrots, and avocado.

3. Tightly roll up the contents in the Nori sheet like a burrito or sushi roll. Seal the end seam with water (or some wasabi paste, if you'd like a little kick!) to hold the roll together.

4. Eat whole like a burrito, or slice the roll into bite-size pieces and enjoy!

ALIVE BREAKFAST CEREAL

Makes 3 servings

In a food processor, blend the following ingredients into a fine meal:

    ¼ cup almonds (soaked overnight to make them easier to digest)

    ¼ cup pumpkin seeds

Empty nut mixture into a bowl. Chop or dice the following ingredients, put in food processor and blend:

    1 pear

    1 apple

    1 cup berries of your choice

Mix all of the ingredients together in a bowl, and top with the following ingredients as garnishes:

    4 de-stemmed figs, rehydrated in water

    ½ teaspoon ginger root, chopped

    Squeeze of lemon

Pinch of pumpkin pie spice
Pinch of Himalayan sea salt
Sprinkle of ground flaxseed, if desired

The Mini-Cleanse

We realize that not everyone has the ability or desire to complete a seven-day cleanse, so here is a regimen that is less extreme yet still very effective if you follow it for at least two or three days. (If you like, you may follow this cleanse for up to seven days.) Remember to drink lots of water and tea.

- Start your morning with a mug of hot water and lemon juice.
- For breakfast (around 8:00 a.m.), enjoy a fresh green juice consisting of celery, cucumber, fennel, rainbow chard or kale, parsley, and apple; or a juice of kale, chard, tomato, carrots, sprouts, and parsley.
- Around 11:00 a.m., enjoy a second green juice.
- At about 12:30 p.m., choose one of the following lunch options:
  - *Option 1*—2 cups of blanched or steamed green leafy veggies or broccoli, cauliflower, spinach, green beans, fennel, cabbage, and zucchini. For the dressing, mix together 3 tablespoons of flax oil and 2 tablespoons of apple cider vinegar or lemon juice, and a pinch of Celtic or Himalayan sea salt. You can add any of these fresh herbs for flavor: parsley, cilantro, mint, tarragon, basil, thyme, ginger, cayenne, and pepper.
  - *Option 2*—A big salad of mixed lettuces such as spinach, arugula, mache (also called lamb's lettuce), and romaine. Be sure to include sprouts (a high-energy food and a great source of protein—sunflower sprouts are especially good). You can also add cucumber, tomato, any of your favorite raw veggies, and your

favorite herbs. Or, try a big salad of fennel, cabbage, and zucchini. (If you're trying to maintain weight, rather than lose it, add half an avocado and 2 tablespoons of sunflower seeds. Use the same dressing as above.)

- Snack a couple of times per day on celery sticks, cucumber slices, or an apple if you feel that you need a little something extra (have no more than one apple per day).
- Drink lots of tea throughout the day and evening, as desired. The best teas for a cleanse include any combination of the following herbs: organic red clover, fennel seed, licorice root, cinnamon bark, alfalfa leaf, gotu kola, English hawthorn berry, cardamom seed, ginger root, burdock root, dandelion root, yellow dock, clove bud, and black pepper. Other choices of tea include peppermint, ginger, chamomile, and dandelion.
- Drink a fizzy, flavored vitamin energy packet such as Aloe C or Oz Effervescent Vitamin C, dissolved in an 8-ounce glass of water.
- Drink a glass of unsweetened cranberry juice diluted with water (one part cranberry juice to two parts water). Add a drop of stevia if you need a little sweetener.
- Drink mineral broth (see recipe on page 33). Make your mineral broth the night before you start your cleanse, as it will last up to three days in the refrigerator.
- Eat your last meal no later than 7:00 p.m., but you can continue drinking teas until bedtime.

Important Cleansing Tips

- Find time to relax.
- Take a hot bath every night with Epsom salts or essential oils.
- Drink your teas.

- Get some light exercise.
- Get thirty minutes of direct sunlight on your body.
- Pamper yourself.
- Get a massage.
- Breathe deeply.
- Stretch.
- Sweat in a sauna or steam room.
- Drink lots of water.
- Be sure to add a system cleanser every day such as Iconic Fizz or Mag-Tea Powder as mentioned earlier.
- Go to sleep early without eating much, and get a good night's rest.
- Take it slowly.

Detox Redux

As with everything else in this book (and in life), there are numerous methods of, and philosophies about, detoxing. So we have included another viewpoint, this one from Dr. Roni DeLuz, a registered nurse with a doctorate in natural health, the founder of the Martha's Vineyard Diet Detox and the author of *21 Pounds in 21 Days*.

Notes from Dr. Roni

Everyone should detox. Detoxing helps flush deadly poisons out of the system, create new healthy cells, keep the arteries clean, eliminate crystalic acids from the joints, eliminate mucus from the digestive system, feed rich minerals to the cells, and increase oxygen in the body. The optimal length of a detox is twenty-one days, which is enough time to allow the body to cleanse major organs.

The principle behind detoxing is simple. When we eat, the body uses a tremendous amount of energy to process and break down the food through the digestive system. When we stop eating, all the energy that previously went into the digestive process now goes toward healing and cleansing. But this is not a starvation diet; it allows you to drink tasty, nutritious cocktails all day, which is great for your energy because the glucose levels in your blood remain stable.

The focus of the Martha's Vineyard Diet Detox is to provide maximum nutrition in small doses throughout the day, feeding the body to create healthy cells while shrinking the body by eliminating waste. Once you feed your body high nutrition and at the same time eliminate waste, your body will begin to shrink fat cells and you will begin to feel a difference.

The type of cleanse I recommend is not only about getting rid of toxins—it's about cellular renewal. That's why I have clients begin their day with a high-ORAC (oxygen radical absorbance capacity) drink made from the powerful antioxidant anthocyanins, known to protect the brain against free radical damage, improve urinary health, and promote healthy liver function. Another morning drink we recommend is made from Essential Greens by Garden Greens, which contains ten green foods including aloe vera gel, Hawaiian blue-green algae, wheat grass, and green tea. (You can find out more about these specific products by visiting Dr. Roni's Web site at www.mvdietdetox.com.)

You would then drink juices every one and a half to two hours throughout the day until 5:00 or 6:00 p.m., when you would have your "soup of the day," made of cooked and blended vegetables and spices of your choosing, using different vegetables every day to provide variety, and adding spices such as garlic, cayenne pepper, curry powder, and no-salt vegetable seasoning.

The philosophy behind this program is to prepare the body for cellular repair with maximum nutrition in small doses, giving the body plenty of opportunity to release toxins along the way. If you want to experience healthy aging, you've got to be aware of everything you put into your body and what it is and isn't doing for you. Only 6 percent of our population reaches the American standards for healthy nutrition—which means that 94 percent doesn't, and that, unfortunately, is reflected in the rising rates of obesity and disease in our country.

There are stages to any cleanse, especially if you've never done one before, or

THE MANY WONDERS
OF DETOX

*I came to the Martha's Vineyard Holistic Retreat in 2006 for a visit just to learn
more about the diet detox program, twenty-one pounds in twenty-one days. I
was tired and depressed and felt I was losing my edge as a lawyer. My body
showed signs of toxicity, as I was emotionally eating everything in sight. Then I consulted with
Dr. Roni, and she educated me on her cleansing detox program, which included ingesting
green juices, berry antioxidants, enzyme-rich juices, live vegetable soups, aloe vera juice, and
herbal supplements. Cleansing my colon and liver was also an integral part of the program. It
changed my life. One amazing benefit (besides the weight loss) was the appearance of my
skin. I noticed that my eyes were brighter, the dark circles under my eyes gradually
disappeared, and the texture of my skin became smoother. Basically, my skin cleared up. From
that point on I changed my lifestyle and have since learned that detoxing also has antiaging
benefits. I was able to regain my muscle mass, and I am now looking good. It's a win-win
situation, and I couldn't feel better.*

THEOPHILUS NIX, JR., FIFTY-THREE,
LAWYER, FATHER OF TWO

if you have a long history of using caffeine, sugar, alcohol, or tobacco. You will
experience varying degrees of withdrawal, and you may feel quite uncomfortable
as you get rid of the substances to which your body is addicted and accustomed.
If you do a seven-day cleanse, the first two or three days may be particularly uncomfortable. Typically, you begin to feel better after the third or fourth day (it
could take longer, depending on the intensity of your addictions).

It's generally best to do a detox program when you have time on your
hands, when you have a light schedule at work, or when you're on vacation.
Once you have experienced such a program and know how your body will
react, you can do a detox at any time. When the week is over, you feel much
lighter. Many people report that they feel much clearer, have a lighter appetite, can manage their blood sugar better, and are better able to control their
cravings. Personally, I always find that my mood is elevated when I complete
a cleanse.

Oz Wraps It Up

As I said at the beginning of this chapter, there are many ways to detox. You don't have to complete a weeklong cleanse. You can modify your diet according to my suggestions on pages 39–40, exercise, get massage work done, or use saunas.

You can also try one of my favorite products, Ultraclear by Metagenics, a food-based powder designed to be consumed in beverage form. Made from rice-protein concentrate, it's used to help the liver perform its detoxifying functions with greater efficiency during a detox program. It's jam-packed with phytonutrients and minerals to protect the liver and promote hepatic antioxidant activity. Because of its unique composition of protein, essential fats in the form of medium-chain triglycerides (MCT), and the right percentage of carbohydrates, it's a perfect meal replacement during a detox program. In addition, it's rich in glutathione (a powerful antioxidant required by the liver to reduce and eliminate toxins) and glutathione precursor nutrients.

I highly endorse detoxification as long as it is done with proper guidance, especially if it's your first time. Many spas, resorts, and ashrams provide their own custom programs, and you may want to take advantage of this service for your first detox. (If you want to experience a really high-end detox, visit the Buchinger Clinic in Germany, famous for its mind-body-spirit weeklong "fasting cure" detoxing program—see the resource guide for contact information.) Or you can ask a local nutritionist, raw food chef, or other health professional with experience in this area to help guide you through the process. If you don't know of anyone, try calling a spa or ashram near your home to find out if they can recommend someone for you.

Over the years, our bodies accumulate all kinds of toxins that build up in our tissues and can harm us later in life. You want to remove these substances as best you can. An effective detox doesn't have to be complicated or prolonged. It can be as simple as having an Ultraclear shake as a breakfast smoothie a few mornings a week, having fresh fruit in the morning, going for a run, or enjoying a sauna. Whatever method you choose, detoxification, though often overlooked, is an important tool in the *Redesigning 50* way of life.

THREE

EATING IN THE REAL WORLD

TIPS FOR DINING OUT

THERE'S ONE THING I want you to understand about nutrition and healthy aging: It's not about following a strict diet or eating only raw food, only protein, only vegetables, or only anything. It's about using the wisdom you've acquired over the years and making smart choices the majority of the time.

It's also about real life and appreciating those things in life that give us pleasure. When, where, and how we dine—and with whom—can add to the stress and discomfort of our lives, or it can give us a break from the hectic pace of everything else we do.

T. S. Wiley, author of *Lights Out: Sleep, Sugar and Survival*, once told me that she considers the breakdown of the traditional family mealtime to be one of the most critical problems our culture faces today. Kids come home from school, prepare their own meals, go to their rooms, and work on their computers. Men and women come home from work, heat something in the microwave, and may or may not have dinner with their spouses. What's been lost is the connection of dining together and the kind of communication that it fosters. This lack of communication only adds to the stress of family life and exacerbates the damaging physical and psychological effects that stress can produce.

In most European countries, families frequently take time to enjoy the dining experience. In restaurants, you will often see extended families—parents, children, grandparents—savoring a meal that may stretch out for more than two or three hours. I would love to see Americans, especially as we age, learn to enjoy fine dining.

If It's Not Pure, It Doesn't Give You Fuel

David Bouley, one of the best-known gourmet chefs in the country, works hard to offer his customers the best-tasting food possible while keeping them healthy. Born and raised in Connecticut, he was strongly influenced by his French heritage and his grandmother's love of cooking. He studied at the Sorbonne and returned to America to work in some of New York's leading restaurants. From 1987 until it closed in 1996, David's own restaurant, Bouley, earned four stars from the *New York Times*. He then opened Bouley Bakery and Danube. Following the tragic events of September 11, 2001, David had to close the two eateries because of their proximity to Ground Zero. However, Danube soon reopened, and Bouley Bakery was relaunched as Bouley.

In 2005, David opened his new Bouley Bakery & Market. He prides himself on finding the best and freshest local ingredients; many of them are for sale in his cellar market, which also houses a cheese room and an area for dry-aging beef. The second floor contains a small sushi bar and a demo kitchen, anchored by a fire engine-red Molteni oven from France.

Everyone deserves to experience the kind of fine dining that Bouley offers, which harks back to European traditions. At this stage of your life, you deserve the best; you deserve to acknowledge and celebrate your accomplishments. One of the things that drew me to David Bouley was his deep understanding and knowledge of the role that food plays in our lives. For years, he has brought traditional French cooking to the United States while traveling the world to learn what global cuisine has to offer. His latest influence is from the Japanese Kaiseki style of cooking.

LESSONS FROM THE MONKS

According to folklore, hundreds of years ago Buddhist priests in strict Zen training used to wrap a hot stone in a towel and place it in their kimono pocket. The heat from the stone would help stave off hunger pangs between the morning and evening meals. The idea was to eat only enough food to sustain themselves for a twenty-four-hour period. "Kaiseki" (literally, stones in the bosom) then came to mean a light meal that is served during a tea ceremony. For many years, Kaiseki cooking was strictly vegetarian, but it now often includes meat, poultry, and seafood as well. Traditional Kaiseki cuisine uses fresh seasonal ingredients and simple seasonings to create dishes that are healthy, flavorful, and beautifully presented.

Notes from David Bouley

When most Americans think of Japanese food, they think only of sushi and sashimi. However, in Japan, sushi and sashimi make up only 10 percent of the menu. The rest is cooked foods, soups, and stews. This is what I have learned over the past several years, working with the prestigious Suji cooking school from Japan. Recently I was privileged to have several Suji instructors visit from Japan with Mr. Suji himself. He's created a very healthy Japanese style of eating that comes from the Kaiseki menu. The main emphasis is on flavor, although every course is designed for its health benefits.

The Suji cooking style combines Kaiseki traditions with principles of nutrition that come from a population-based study of the elderly in Okinawa, Japan. The study began in 1976, after the Japan Ministry of Health, Labor and Welfare confirmed initial reports of outstanding health and long life in Okinawa. Studies showed that the Okinawans' diet included low-fat, water-rich, and high-fiber foods such as sweet potatoes, vegetables, whole grains, fruits, soy foods, and other beans and fish, with limited amounts of lean meats. Although the diet contains a fair amount of carbohydrates, it also contains about half the caloric density (or calories per gram of food) of the American diet.

Japanese people go to a Kaiseki restaurant for special occasions. If you need to entertain a special guest, Kaiseki is a good choice. A Kaiseki meal consists of several small dishes and often includes a salad, sliced raw fish, tempura, grilled fish, miso soup, rice, asparagus tips paired with smoked salmon, and pureed chestnuts.

My training in French and Japanese cuisines has taught me to use only the best ingredients. If it's not pure, it's not going to give you energy or true satisfaction. Purity of the food is what gives people the most enjoyment. For instance, consider the following two ways that people can eat chocolate. If I give one person a chocolate sundae jam-packed with cheap ingredients and lots of sugar, and another person half an ounce of high-quality chocolate with a high level of cacao, they'll have very different experiences. The first person will have to dig and dig through the sundae for the satisfaction he's never going to get, while the other person will savor every little bite of the chocolate and end up feeling fulfilled.

What I care about most is the nutritional value of food. I am now learning more about the science of food, nutrition, and diet. In my collaboration with Oz, he teaches me how people should eat to be healthy, and I teach him how to make it taste good. My goal is to bring the flavor forward without distraction, obtain clarity in taste and presentation, and ultimately allow the diner to fully realize the essence of the ingredients, calling forth natural flavors in a healthful cuisine. I don't necessarily have all the answers, but I know that we can make healthy food that tastes incredible.

ARE YOU EATING MORE NOW AND ENJOYING IT LESS?

If so, you're not alone. According to a survey conducted by the Pew Research Center in April 2006, 59 percent of Americans say they eat more than they should. However, just 39 percent of the adults surveyed say they enjoy eating "a great deal," down from the 48 percent who said the same thing in a Gallup poll survey in 1989.

The survey also found a correlation between stress and eating (to most of us, this comes as no surprise). Of those who said they frequently felt stressed, 21 percent reported they often overate, and 25 percent said they ate too much junk food. Of those who said they hardly ever felt stressed, 15 percent reported they often overate, and 15 percent said they ate too much junk food. For most of the people in the survey (73 percent), convenience was the top reason for eating junk food, with another 24 percent reporting that it was because junk food was more affordable.

A Simpler Approach to Food

Whenever people start on a diet or any kind of nutritional program, one of the first things they ask is "What do I do when I eat out?" Eating out is a great American pastime, and you don't have to give it up to maintain a healthy lifestyle. It helps when there are restaurateurs like Gennaro Sbarro around.

Sbarro hails from the legacy of the Sbarro Italian Eateries, found in malls worldwide. The company operates more than 950 Sbarro Italian Eateries in forty-eight states and thirty-two countries. Gennaro knew at a young age that he wanted to continue the family tradition. In January 2005, Gennaro left the family business to embark on his own culinary ventures, including opening Salute!, an upscale Italian/Mediterranean restaurant on Madison Avenue in the heart of Manhattan. The menu has been designed to introduce top specialty dishes from all regions of Italy, Mediterranean delights, and healthy gourmet fare.

When I was introduced to Gennaro, I knew immediately that we were simpatico. He and I are both interested in fostering delicious dining that is healthful as well. Consequently, we decided to collaborate on the menu for his new restaurant, and it contains several dishes based on the Mediterranean diet

49

that I recommend for patrons who want to enjoy guilt-free, mouth-watering dishes.

Notes from Gennaro Sbarro

My training and background have helped me develop a simpler approach to food. Simple ingredients such as olive oil, tomatoes, and fresh vegetables make wonderful, flavorful dishes that don't have to be drenched in butters and creams or be served with a heavy steak. It's the quality of the ingredients that makes a meal flavorful, enjoyable, and healthy. When you eat a simple fish salad, a simple tomato salad, or a simple dish with plum tomatoes and pasta, you feel good afterward. You don't feel heavy and weighed down. At Salute! I aim to simplify the life and cuisine of the restaurant so that people can have a healthier dining experience while enjoying the essential flavors of the foods they're eating. The dishes are never overly complex or full of chemicals, preservatives, or harmful elements.

Every day we take steps to incorporate more organic sauces, organic tomatoes, and vegetables in our cooking. Since the restaurant has been open, we've made significant strides in finding the right quality and flavor of organic products to replace what we had been buying. On my menu, we even have some starred choices—dishes that Oz and I have determined to be the healthier-choice items.

People often think that in an Italian restaurant they're going to get a heavy meal, not necessarily a healthy one. But consumers in the United States and abroad have become more health conscious, and so have we. I've had the good fortune in my life to open restaurants around the world, and I've watched eating habits change over the course of twenty years. For example, for many years, fried calzones (Italian turnovers made of pizza dough and stuffed with cheese, meat, and/or vegetables) were one of the most popular items in Sbarro's restaurants. When I was young, I ate fried-dough calzones on a regular basis, and I remember feeling heavy and sleepy afterward. Sbarro's still sells them today, but they now account for an insignificant portion of sales. Years ago, most of the items on the menu would be pasta with heavy sauces, meatballs, and sausage. Now, salads make up a significant section of the menu. Since the restaurant first opened, we've doubled the number of salads on the menu.

As a restaurateur, I know that customers can sometimes be reluctant to ask for food to be prepared a particular way, to substitute an item on the menu, or to hold the breadbasket. We don't want our customers to feel that way. Therefore, we offer nutritionally sound choices on the menu and are pleased to serve meals that keep our customers healthy and happy.

ANOTHER REASON TO EAT MEDITERRANEAN STYLE

In April 2006, a study published in the *Annals of Neurology* claimed that people who ate a Mediterranean diet had a 40 percent lower risk of developing Alzheimer's disease than those who ate the conventional American diet. Dr. Nikolaos Scarmeas, assistant professor of neurology at Columbia University Medical Center and leader of the study, explained that it's the Mediterranean diet as a whole, not any one particular element, that is beneficial. Theories about why it works say that the benefit could be due to its effect on blood vessels, reducing the risk of blockage, or that the foods in the diet are rich in antioxidants, or that the diet reduces the amount of inflammation in the body.

Oz Wraps It Up

I believe that our diets should be healthy but as nonrestrictive as possible. Therefore, I would never say that we should eat only Mediterranean-style or Japanese-style cooking. Of course, there are examples of healthy eating styles everywhere in the world. No matter where you're eating out, you can almost always choose seafood or ask for lean meat that is baked or broiled (rather than fried), and lots of vegetables. And go somewhere that serves managed portions instead of serving sizes large enough to feed your whole family. Look for quality and freshness over quantity. Eateries that offer organic foods are a good choice. Wherever you live, you should be able to find exciting, entertaining restaurants that serve regional and seasonal foods—foods that are grown in your area and vary with the seasons.

REJUVE-NATION:

FEELING LIKE THIRTY AGAIN

*"Youth would be an ideal state if
it came a little later in life."*

—HERBERT HENRY ASQUITH,
BRITISH PRIME MINISTER, 1908–1916

THERE ISN'T MUCH we can do about getting older. Every creature on earth ages with every passing day. Even though we can't alter our chronology, we can change *the way we age*. In Part I of this book, we discussed how food-as-fuel can help keep our bodies running at peak efficiency even as we get older. In Part II, we focus on rejuvenation—the phenomenon of restoring vitality and freshness to the aging body.

What happens to our bodies as we age? Unfortunately, by the time we reach the age of thirty-five, most of our systems begin to decline, with the first signs often appearing in the musculoskeletal system. We lose 4 to 6 percent of our muscle mass for every decade of our lives after the age of forty. Our eyesight begins to decline, and many forty-year-olds find that they can't read the small print (or any print at all) without reading glasses. As we get into our fifties, many of us experience varying degrees of hearing loss. We even lose taste buds as we age, so that many foods begin to taste bitter or bland. Weight gain is another factor of aging. As we get older, the proportion of body fat to muscle increases by more than 30 percent. We lose subcutaneous fat (fat beneath the skin), which increases wrinkling, and we gain fat in the abdominal area.

Our internal organs also decline. In most cases, the decline itself is not dramatic enough to do us harm, but it does make us more vulnerable to environmental factors, toxins, and illness. The immune system produces fewer antibodies, so infections can be more frequent and more severe. Blood sugar levels rise faster after eating, which makes us prone to diabetes. Our calcium absorption decreases, which increases the chances of osteoporosis. In men, the prostate enlarges and testosterone decreases, which causes urinary retention and erectile dysfunction. Women lose estrogen and are at increased risk for coronary artery disease (not to mention hot flashes and mood swings). The heart muscle cannot pump as strenuously as it once did, so we cannot perform physically the way we did in our youth. And last but not least, blood flow to the brain decreases, and nerve impulses are transmitted less efficiently, which means slower reflexes and reduced mental functioning.

Depressing? It need not be. While we can't stop the natural effects of many decades of wear and tear on the body, the fact is that more people are aging "successfully" than ever before—which means they are getting older without experiencing debilitating disease and disability. Every year the average life span for men and women is increasing. And more and more people are discovering ways of living their later years with a youthful vitality that was unheard of just a few decades ago.

That's what this section is all about. We can reduce, delay, and ameliorate the natural declines of aging by addressing two important factors: flexibility and stress. Increasing flexibility and decreasing stress constitute a sure recipe for rejuvenating the body and the mind.

Focus on Flexibility

There are many different kinds of stress in our lives; some are mental, others physical. As we age, it becomes increasingly important to address both kinds of stress equally. Flexibility helps us sustain or increase our mobility and with-stand bodily stress without injury. Flexibility can also help reduce stress and promote a greater sense of well-being.

The older we get, the more important it is to keep moving. A sedentary life can accelerate the natural loss of muscle mass and further slow the already slowed response time of our muscles. With age, our tendons (the cordlike tissues that attach muscles to bones) lose water and stiffen, becoming less able to absorb stress. We also lose tissue and mineral content in our bones, making them fragile and prone to osteoporosis. Cartilage (which provides cushioning between the bones) and ligaments (connective tissues between bones) become less elastic, making our joints prone to arthritis and reducing flexibility.

In the February 7, 2003, issue of the *AAOS Bulletin*, the American Academy of Orthopaedic Surgeons stated that "Many of the changes in our musculoskeletal system result more from disuse than from simple aging. Fewer than 10 percent of Americans participate in regular exercise, and the most sedentary group is over age 50." It has been proved that we can counteract these declining natural processes by working to improve flexibility through exercise. This doesn't necessarily mean we have to take aerobics classes three times a week, but it does call for moderate amounts of physical activity, including weight training to increase muscle mass and strength. Later in this section, we discuss ways to keep the body strong and flexible throughout the second half of life.

De-stress Versus Distress

While flexibility can help us deal with physical stress, we also need to decrease the amount of mental stress in our lives (or at least find better ways of coping with it). We modern-day *Homo sapiens* spend much of our lives in distress—our lives are filled with strain, anxiety, and suffering. And for many people in our pressure-filled world, life is one big stress-filled event. In fact, many people don't really have the mechanism for dealing with stress on a daily basis but rather have geared themselves up to perform primarily in the presence of enormous stress. This may have helped them attain huge success in their fields, but long hours of work, lack of sleep, and even hormonal changes all contribute to problems with weight, energy, mood, and on-the-job performance. We need to find ways to deal with the years of unremitting stress on our bodies.

Stress is often the cause of physical pain and discomfort. Unfortunately, it can also be the cause of a weakened immune system—another symptom of aging. When you address the problems of stress, using methods such as exercise, yoga, and massage (discussed further in the following chapters), you also improve your immunological profile. One way to do this is to visit a spa to give yourself a chance to relax, and to learn to bring the spa experience home to continue the relaxation process.

CORTISOL: THE STRESS HORMONE

Hormones, those powerful little chemicals produced by glands in the body, circulate in the bloodstream. They control growth and development, reproduction, sexual characteristics, and blood sugar levels, and they influence the way the body uses and stores energy. Cortisol, a hormone produced in the adrenal gland, is critical to the body's ability to mediate stress. Cortisol allows us to respond to any kind of stress—be it a dangerous situation, a personal tragedy, an illness, a high-powered business deal, or a screaming three-year-old. As we age, the systems that regulate these stress hormones become compromised and impaired. While we may produce the same amount of cortisol we always have (if not more), it simply doesn't work as efficiently as it used to.

High levels of cortisol are a main factor in the loss of muscle and the accumulation of fat, especially around the stomach and gut area. Many studies have shown the deleterious effects of too much cortisol. "Cortisol Effects on Body Mass, Blood Pressure, and Cholesterol in the General Population" (Robert Fraser and Mary C. Ingram, et al., *Hypertension* 33, 1999: 1364–68) showed that there is a correlation between high cortisol levels and higher blood pressure, body mass, and cholesterol. Excess cortisol is also harmful to brain cells. A study titled "Decreased Memory Performance in Healthy Humans Induced by Stress-Level Cortisol Treatments" (John W. Newcomer and Gregg Selke, et al., *Archives of General Psychiatry* 56, 1999: 527–33) showed that exposure to high doses of cortisol can "decrease specific elements of memory performance in otherwise healthy individuals." This is apparently even worse for women. "The Relationship between Stress Induced Cortisol Levels and Memory Differs Between Men and Women" (Oliver T. Wolf and Nicole C. Schommer, et al., *Psychoneuroendocrinology* 26, 2001: 711–20) states that "Epidemiological as well as experimental studies in elderly subjects have suggested that postmenopausal women are more susceptible to the memory impairing effects of elevated cortisol levels than elderly men."

All this means that as we get older it is more important than ever to modify our lifestyles to inhibit the production of too much cortisol. In other words, chill out!

FOUR

THE SPA EXPERIENCE

A WEEK AWAY OR AN EVENING AT HOME

SOMETIMES WHAT YOU need most to rejuvenate yourself is a break—a change of routine, a vacation from responsibilities, a chance to be pampered and indulged. Whether you go for a day, a week, or a weekend, a spa can be a great place to unwind in an environment geared toward fitness, healthy eating, relaxation, and renewal. Many different kinds of spas can be found around the country, offering a variety of services. There are spas that focus on weight loss, spas that address particular medical concerns, spas that offer outdoor experiences like rock climbing and hiking, spas that feature special services and body treatments like mud baths or hot water pools, and spas that take you on spiritual journeys through meditation, yoga, and tai chi. Many spas offer combinations of the above. If you plan to visit a spa, do your homework and choose one that suits your interests, offers the programs and services you're looking for, is easily accessible, and falls within your budget.

Not so long ago, a spa was a luxury meant only for the rich and famous. But these days, the spa experience is really an essential component of a healthy lifestyle. Yes, some spas are very expensive, but others are not. There are now day spas that offer single services and affordable packages. And, as discussed later in this chapter, you can give yourself a relaxing, invigorating spa experience right in the comfort of your own home. Taking time for yourself becomes even more important as you age; the mind, body, and spirit need the opportunity to rejuvenate. A visit to a spa or a spa treatment at home can help release toxins, refresh your mind, and recharge your batteries. It is a chance to de-stress and enjoy a few hours of restful pampering.

Sometimes, however, the only way to get both your mind and your body into a more receptive zone for making a new start on life is to take yourself out of your environment—get off the phone, get away from workaholic triggers, and relieve yourself of your day-to-day responsibilities. In this chapter, you'll learn about three of the best spas in the country. Two of them are "sleep-away" spas, where you can enjoy several days of rest and peace. One is a day spa that offers a midweek respite from the daily grind. You'll hear from Erica Zack, assistant director, and Diane Allan, fitness training coordinator, at the Golden Door Spa in California about what the spa experience means. You'll also learn about Miraval, the spa and resort set in the incredible environment of the Arizona desert, and Cornelia Day Resort, one of the newest day spas to hit the Big Apple.

61

Notes from Erica Zack on Entering the Golden Door

Located in Escondido, California, about forty miles northeast of San Diego, the Golden Door spa and fitness resort takes its inspiration from ancient Japanese Honjin inns in its architecture and philosophy and is legendary for its care and service to guests. Guests stay in rooms with private patios surrounded by meticulously landscaped courtyards of camellia bushes, koi ponds or sand gardens, and antique Japanese art. The spa serves gourmet meals made with fresh ingredients from the Golden Door's own organic garden.

Not so long ago we thought of a spa as a place for only the very pampered. Now we think of it as an investment in preventive health. Genetics and advances in science and technology now enable most of us to live into our eighties and beyond. It's important to invest our money in things and practices that contribute to our mental and physical health. We must take very good care of ourselves, especially as we get older.

One thing we must focus on is stress management. We know so much more these days about how stress affects our health—85 percent, if not more, of all medical illness has some derivation in stress. Recent advances in MRI (magnetic resonance imaging) technology have allowed doctors to see tangible changes in our brains when we release—or don't release—stress hormones. This is no longer considered just a new-age concept. Even the corporate world has jumped on board; in fact, some companies offer their employees perks like massages because they recognize that employees who are less stressed and more present tend to be happier and more productive.

If you want to look and feel naturally younger, it's not necessary to use invasive methods like facelifts or buy into the starvation mentality to get as thin as possible. You don't just want to look good; you want to be functional, too. You want to be strong with flexibility and endurance, but endurance has to be built. And going to a spa regularly, or even frequently, can help you understand and achieve this kind of strength on a deeper level. A good spa creates a very safe environment that dismantles the walls of your everyday stress and enables you to reconnect with the wisdom of your body.

For instance, I teach a class here called Kaizen, which is a Japanese philosophy that is used to improve corporate productivity, but which we apply here to behavior change. The word *Kaizen* means "continuous improvement" and comes from the Japanese words *Kai,* meaning school, and *Zen,* meaning wisdom. It's a philosophy of implementing change without regard for time or speed—taking baby steps toward a goal without time pressures. In our Western society, we are trained to think that if improvement is not huge or dramatic, it somehow doesn't count. This mentality is a setup for failure. The goal of Kaizen is to move from one small step to the next without becoming consumed by the whole, until eventually you can look back and say, "Look at all that I've accomplished!"

Notes from Diane Allan

Shortly after a guest's arrival at the Golden Door, he or she has an interview to discuss goals as well as any medical restrictions so that we can customize his or her schedule. Besides wanting to reduce stress, many guests want to lose weight and improve their overall fitness. A new lecture titled "Optimizing Weight Management through Exercise," presented by fitness director Trish Martin, gives detailed information on how to reduce body fat, increase lean muscle tissue, and effectively manage weight. Some of the main points discussed are varying intensity levels and types of cardiovascular exercises. For example, if walking is a preferred activity, a person can walk a moderate pace two to three times per week and do a more challenging walk or interval training (alternating high intensity with light-to-moderate) one to two times per week. On the other days, the person can go for a light-intensity level walk or use that day for rest.

Ideally, it is best to vary the types of cardiovascular exercise. This helps prevent boredom, burnout, and injuries. In addition, different muscles are used for different activities, which helps achieve greater results. Suggestions for cardiovascular exercise include bicycling, swimming, walking, running, hiking, aerobic dance, water aerobics, and use of the machines such as elliptical trainers, treadmills, and stair masters.

For weight loss, an individual should gradually work up to 45 to 90 minutes of cardiovascular exercise most days of the week. The exercise can be done at one time during the day or in two to three mini-workouts throughout the day.

For effective weight management, it is important to increase lean muscle mass by doing resistance training two to three times per week. This can be done with strength-training machines, dumbbells, tubing, elastic bands, or body weight exercises (push-ups, squats, etc.). Increasing lean muscle mass will help raise one's resting metabolic rate so that more calories are burned per day.

63

The Miracle of Miraval, Life in Balance

One of the most luxurious spas in this country is Miraval, Life in Balance®, located in Catalina, Arizona, in the middle of the Sonoran Desert. The programs and activities at Miraval all revolve around a central philosophy that they call "mindfulness." When you learn to appreciate the moment you're in—rather than worry about the past or the future—life gets better. There is no strict regimen and no pressure. Guests are free to create daily agendas that suit their whims, goals, and moods.

In September 2005, Miraval announced the appointment of Dr. Andrew Weil, author of several bestsellers including *8 Weeks to Optimum Health,* as director of integrative health and healing.

Many activities at Miraval are designed to help guests challenge their comfort zones, including nighttime rock climbing, walking along a log thirty feet above the ground, and climbing a shaky twenty-five-foot wooden pole and then jumping off.

For many people, however, the experience is more about the opportunity to let go, calm down, and enjoy a change from their usual urban environment. Often, they begin every day with a nature walk in the desert and learn to appreciate the clean mountain air, the sun beating down, the stars at night, and the rare opportunity to admire the saguaro cactus and unusual boulder formations.

While at Miraval, guests can also schedule massage and bodywork, customized to their needs and special problems. Many people rave about the Thai massage, a technique that incorporates yoga stretches with gentle pressure along energy lines. Thai massage is great for increasing flexibility, relieving muscle and joint tension, stimulating internal organs, and balancing the body's energy flow.

A Day at Cornelia

If you can't get away for a full week or even a long weekend, you might try visiting a day spa for some instant mind/body/spirit rejuvenation. A day spa can be a stand-alone facility, part of a hotel or resort complex, or an adjunct to a health club. These spas usually offer a variety of services from which you can choose just one or two (like a massage and/or a facial) or pamper yourself with a whole day's worth.

One of the most prestigious of these day spas is Cornelia Day Resort in New York City. The spa was founded by Cornelia Zicu, a Romanian refugee who has translated her grandmother's natural beauty treatments into a line of high-end products and has become a world-renowned skin-care expert. The foundation of all of Cornelia's products and treatments at the spa is an extract of mineral-rich mud taken from Lake Amara in Romania.

There is nothing more relaxing than interrupting a busy schedule for a day of treatments at Cornelia, beginning with the Romanian mud bath (concentrated extracts are infused into the bath water so that you get the benefits without actually having to bathe in mud) and continuing to exfoliation and a stimulating body massage.

"The minerals in the bath draw the blood to the surface of the skin and get it pumping," says Cornelia. "Skin gets dry and old-looking for many reasons, including the fact that as you age, the blood pumps less oxygen and fewer nutrients to the surface. The skin doesn't have the energy to regenerate that it had when you were young. Every once in a while, you need to give it a little help."

You can also try Cornelia's signature Microablation and Tri-phasic facials. The Microablation is a combination of saline and radio waves that create a plasma field that permeates the skin to stimulate collagen production and cell renewal. This is followed by the Tri-phasic electropulse facial, which uses electric frequency to activate the muscles of the skin.

65

Here's what happens when you spend a day at a spa: you forget about everyone and everything. It's like taking a long winter's nap. You're completely relaxed. Nothing but you matters. It's nice to take a break from everybody else and just be into yourself, even if it's only for a day.

The Spa Experience at Home

As you get older, it becomes more and more important to take time for yourself. Indulge yourself once in a while—or more often if possible. If you don't have the time or the budget to go to a spa, you can create a spa experience for yourself at home, even if only for a few hours. Decide whether you want to do it alone or with friends. Give yourself a manicure, a pedicure, or a facial. Hire someone to give you a massage at home, or if you're with friends, give each other massages. Turn off the phones, the computer, and the television, and create a spot for quiet meditation. Light candles. Take a long bath with soft lighting, soothing scents, and beauty products.

Tips for Setting Up a Day Spa at Home

- *Set the Mood with Scent*: There are thousands of scented candles and essential oils on the market today that can fill a room with wonderful aromas such as cinnamon, rose, lavender, eucalyptus, sage, jasmine, and citrus. Keep a variety on hand so that you can change the scent as you change your mood. The flickering glow of candles is also calming and relaxing.
- *Indulge in Do-It-Yourself Spa Treatments*: Try your own water therapy. Exfoliate with a gentle body scrubber to remove dry skin and stimulate circulation, then relax in a nice warm tub. You can buy relatively inexpensive appliances to turn your tub into a whirlpool, or simply use foaming bath gel to give your spirits a lift.
- *Soothe Your Savage Beast*: Fill your room or house with music that you find particularly relaxing. This can work wonders to help stop the "chatter" that sometimes clutters your mind when you're trying to unwind. Or you might try something revolutionary: silence! Sometimes you just need a quiet space of your own to sort out your thoughts and let your mind drift wherever it wants to go. As the psychiatrist and author Elisabeth Kübler-Ross said in her book *The Tunnel and the Light*, "There is no need to go to India or anywhere else to find peace. You will find that deep place of silence right in your room, your garden or even your bathtub."

The Massage Experience: Releasing Mind and Body

One of the main reasons people go to spas is to get massages. One of the oldest and simplest forms of therapy, massage is a system of stroking, pressing, and kneading different areas of the body to relieve pain and to relax, stimulate, and tone the body. Among the many types of massage are Swedish, Thai, deep tissue, hot stone, and shiatsu.

Studies indicate that massage is critical for decreasing anxiety and calming respiratory rates in people who are under tremendous stress. One study showed that premature babies and infants who were massaged gained more weight and fared better than children who were not. Massage therapy has well-documented positive effects on the immune system. Research has shown that office workers who get massages regularly are more alert and perform better than people who don't. Massage has been shown to reduce the heart rate, lower blood pressure, relax muscles, improve range of motion, decrease anxiety, and increase endorphins (which is why you feel so good afterward). Massage is also very effective in postoperative and postinjury rehabilitation.

You don't have to go to a spa for the massage experience. There are massage therapists all over the country. Some have their own studios, and others will bring their own table and come right to your home. Finding a good massage therapist is often a matter of trial and error. Some specialize in a particular type of massage, while others provide a combination of many types. You may find that you like the kind of massage that really "works you over" and is actually painful but leaves you feeling wonderful after it's done. Or you may prefer a more gentle massage that relaxes you so much it may even put you to sleep.

"No two clients react the same way," says massage therapist Sheila Wormer. She explains:

Some are quiet the whole time and say nothing. Others talk through the whole massage and reveal secrets they have told no one else. Some people laugh; some people cry. Whatever the reaction, the massage helps them release—not just body tension, but mental tension as well. It's a healing exercise, like yoga. Massage opens you up, from the outside in. It's all connected. If one part of your body isn't working right, the rest of your body tries to compensate. It's as if you have ten people pulling on a rope and one of them falls down or lets go. The person nearest the one who gave up has to work harder, which affects the next person. It's a chain reaction. So if you can release the areas of greatest tension, it will have positive effects on the entire body.

Massage therapist Maria Alonso adds that bodywork benefits not only the muscles but the mind as well:

It puts you in a state of mind where you're more at ease, less stressed. Emotions can actually be stored in your muscles; holding in that emotion causes much of the physical tension we experience. And stress is a known factor of aging. That's why massage is important for anyone who wants to slow down the aging process.

Massage is passive-active exercising. In other words, the therapist is working your muscles for you. Massage works to tone and stimulate all systems of the body. It helps to tone muscle; that's why it's especially good for older people who perhaps don't get as much exercise as they used to. It's good for the cardiovascular system. And because you're stimulating the adipose tissue, you're stimulating the fat cells to burn. It also helps you look younger—for instance, if you massage your face every morning, you help to rejuvenate the skin by bringing the blood supply to the surface, giving you the rosy glow of youth.

Oz Wraps It Up

In any age-reversal program, the management of stress is critical. Stress, as we all know, comes in many different guises—from minor stresses caused by daily annoyances to major stresses caused by family, relationship, or career issues and illness or injury, that erode our stability, corrupt our health, and make us age more quickly. The stress-related disorders that we experience with age can in many instances be undone, reversed, or slowed by occasional pampering. Visit a spa for a week, a weekend, or a single day. Get a massage on a regular basis. Set aside a quiet hour for yourself without e-mail, phone calls, or family interruptions. You'll be amazed at what these breaks in routine can do for you, even in the most stressful times.

FIVE

TRAINING FOR LIFE

GET YOUR BODY MOVING

WE LIVE IN a sedentary world. If we're not sitting on the couch watching television, we're sitting at a desk working on the computer. We hardly have to get up anymore. We can shop for nearly anything without moving more than a finger. At home we have remote controls for almost every appliance we own. At work we no longer have to get out of our chairs to reach for the dictionary or encyclopedia—we can access the dictionary and Wikipedia on line. We don't even have to get up to answer the phone; it travels with us wherever we go.

All this technology and convenience may have made us a more advanced society, but it has also helped make us overweight and prone to disease. We all know that exercise is good for us, but just in case you had any doubts about what exercise can do for you, here are a few reminders:

- *Exercise Reduces the Risk of Heart Disease:* In recent years, the emphasis has been on foods that keep your heart healthy. However, exercise is just as important as food, if not more so, in reducing heart disease. Studies have shown that levels of physical activity are much more closely related to risk of death from heart disease than the food you eat. One reason is that the heart is a muscle, and when a muscle is not exercised it can become flaccid and weak. The heart requires exercise to work effectively and efficiently and to maintain its endurance and ability to circulate blood through the body.

- *Exercise Reduces the Risk of Breast Cancer:* A study conducted by the Keck School of Medicine of the University of Southern California and published in the November 2005 issue of the *Journal of the National Cancer Institute* linked physical activity to a lower risk of breast cancer and proposed several mechanisms whereby exercise might be effective. First, exercise can lower the blood levels of female hormones, particularly estrogen and progesterone, not only in adolescents and young adults but even in postmenopausal women. Researchers believe that higher circulating levels of female hormones may raise the risk of breast cancer by stimulating breast cells to divide and multiply. Second, women who exercise regularly also appear to be more sensitive to insulin and to have lower levels of insulin in their blood. A study conducted by the Fred Hutchinson Research Center and published in the *Cancer Research* journal showed that overweight older women can reduce unhealthy estrogen levels and their risk of breast cancer by decreasing fat through exercise. The study showed that a group of women, ages fifty to seventy-five, significantly lowered their levels of estrogen when assigned to a program of moderate exercise. Several studies have also shown that exercise also reduces the risks of other cancers, including prostate and colon cancer, although the reasons are not yet known.

- *Exercise May Delay or Prevent Memory Loss and Dementia:* We naturally lose a certain amount of mental ability as we age. But, according to a study in the September 2005 *Journal of Neuroscience*, exercise may delay or even reverse age-associated memory loss. The study showed that mice that started exercising in old age were better able to learn new tasks and had more message-relaying neurons in the brain than did their sedentary counterparts. Other studies have shown that exercise may help ward off dementia among older people—especially those who participate in a variety of activities, such as aerobics and gardening—the theory being that taking part in different activities keeps more parts of the brain functioning.

In this chapter we hear from several exercise experts, including meditation and yoga teacher and ordained swami Robin Cofer, and three excellent trainers: Oscar Smith (personal trainer to supermodels and celebrities, including Petra Nemcova, Rosario Dawson, and Ed Burns, and founder of O-Diesel personal fitness studio), fitness guru David Barton (owner of David Barton gyms), and Suzanne Meth (client services manager for Equinox at Columbus Circle in New York City).

Redesigning Exercise

Just as I would like to change the emphasis from regimented diets to making smart food choices one meal at a time, I would also like to change the way we think about exercise. Most of us think of exercise as a jog in the park, a run on the treadmill, or an aerobics class at the gym. But exercise takes many forms, and one of my favorite forms is yoga.

While yoga is helpful to people of all ages, it is especially beneficial as you get older because it stretches the body, tones the muscles, and relaxes the mind. Much of the practice of yoga focuses on the spine, the support structure and command center that stretches throughout your entire body. Yoga helps you develop a stronger, more flexible, better aligned, and healthier spine.

Yoga, which originated in India and dates back more than five thousand years, has been defined as "the control of activities of one's mind." Through the practice of yoga, an individual can gain knowledge about physical, emotional, mental, and spiritual well-being. Yoga provides a multitude of benefits, such as the following:

- Reduces respiratory problems, including asthma
- Decreases high blood pressure
- Reduces stress and tension

71

WALKING TALL

Exercising has changed for me over the years. When I was young, I went to the gym and took aerobic classes, but I got tired from it and tired of it. I haven't done that for many years. Now I walk, I swim, and I do yoga. I live in an area that's very beautiful and very hilly. So my walks are actually quite strenuous.

But about twenty years ago, I got into yoga. Yoga is wonderful. First of all, it's weight bearing. You just feel so strong after a tough yoga class. It strengthens my muscles and helps me be able to walk farther and swim better. It's also great for flexibility, and to me, flexibility is the key to everything, especially as you get older. It keeps joints flexible. It's incredible to do a forward bend and really take your time doing it and feel every part of you go into it. Even though it's sometimes hard to hold a position, and even though there are so many different poses to learn, I think yoga is the most complete type of exercise program out there in terms of what it does for your body. And it's something you can do throughout your whole life, no matter how old you are.

Yoga makes you so aware of your body and your posture—even if you're walking, just thinking about doing a backbend opens up your whole chest. You actually feel taller. Another good thing is that you can always fit yoga into your life. You don't have to be in a class. I get up in the morning and do half an hour or forty minutes of going through a series of stretches and poses. It's a great way to start the day. And if you're traveling, you can get up and do fifteen minutes of yoga, and you feel great.

I do a little bit each day, but I fit it into my day, even if it's late at night or early in the morning. It's become part of my routine, like brushing my teeth. That's what I love about it—you can fit it in whenever it works for you. You can get a great workout without having to drive to the gym and do two hours of cycling and jumping up and down.

RICKI LUBART, FIFTY-ONE,
MARRIED, MOTHER

- Reduces anxiety and depression
- Provides pain relief
- Helps reduce and prevent back pain
- Provides relief from arthritis
- Increases overall endurance and energy levels
- Improves balance and flexibility

- Eases chronic insomnia
- Enhances mental performance
- Aids detoxification and flushing out of toxins

For me, yoga is primarily about flexibility and breathing. Because of the flexibility and toning achievable in yoga, it has become an option for women who are suffering from or concerned about osteoporosis. We know that osteoporosis can be prevented and treated through regular weight-bearing exercise; yoga is an excellent low-impact, weight-bearing exercise that stimulates bone building for both the upper body and the lower body.

Proper breathing, which is also central to yoga, is all too rare in our society of shallow breathers. Our bodies are often constricted and tight from anxiety, stress, and fear. Yoga helps us control our breathing to increase the flow of oxygen to the blood and the brain and to strengthen *prana*, our vital life energy.

Notes from Robin Cofer on Yoga

There are many reasons to practice yoga, but for me one of the most important is that it gives you a great sense of well-being. Yoga affects the entire system, physiologically and psychologically—body, mind, and soul. Most people don't realize that yoga is a science, not some kind of pseudoreligion. Western science is trying to catch up to what the yogis have known for thousands of years about the human body.

The other reason to practice yoga is for flexibility. Many people find that the older they get, the tighter their joints and muscles become. Yoga helps loosen those areas, which translates into an easier time moving around in the world, such as simply getting up from a chair or in and out of a car—the small things that can be so frustrating and stressful.

Yoga is all about creating space. You want to create space between the skin and the bones and the muscles so that you feel extended, not all scrunched up. These days, most people walk around hunched over from sitting too long at the computer, in front of the TV, or in cars and airplanes. Yoga opens you up and elongates the spine. For women who are in their forties and fifties, yoga is a perfect weight-bearing exercise. It also teaches balance, which is essential as you get older so that you don't fall and break any fragile bones. That's the physical part of yoga. The psychological part of yoga is about creating space between thoughts, which is achieved through meditation.

There are many different types of yoga. The most popular type, the one that's taught in most gyms and studios, is hatha yoga, which is usually fairly slow-paced and gentle and can provide a good introduction to the basic yoga poses. I teach kundalini yoga, which emphasizes breathwork in conjunction with physical movement in order to free energy in the lower body and allow it to move upward. Kundalini often uses rapid, repetitive movements, but can also involve holding poses for an extended amount of time, and the teacher will often lead the class in call-and-response chanting. Kundalini yoga incorporates conscious, intense breathwork to oxygenate the body to the hilt. Many people compare the resulting high with that of a fantastic run.

Every form of yoga affects your internal organs through the bending and twisting of your body. In this way, yoga can also help you detoxify; whenever you twist, the liver and other internal organs release toxins. The best thing about yoga is that it's good for everyone, no matter what your shape or age. One of my students started when she was seventy-five years old. When she began, she could barely bend over, and now she can touch her palms flat to the floor. Yoga is so adaptable that even people in wheelchairs can practice it because there are so many things you can do with the upper body.

Yoga is particularly good for anyone who is always on the go (and aren't we all?), whether you're a stay-at-home mom or dad or a high-powered executive. Yoga allows you to reconnect with your breath, which calms you down. Many people take shallow breaths from their chests and are really disconnected from their core. In yoga, you breathe from your center. Think about it: You take your shallowest breaths when you're frightened or anxious. Really shallow chest breathing is anxiety driven. So just slowing down and deeply connecting to your breath allows you to reduce your anxiety—and therefore your cortisol levels—and gives your entire system a chance to rejuvenate. People in this country don't know how to relax, and that ages them prematurely. One of the best things you can do for yourself every day is to stop what you're doing for five minutes and simply take five deep breaths. This will center you and allow you to move on with your day. A successful meditation—and this means quality of time, not quantity—will reset your mind, your mood, and your heart rate.

Getting to the Gym

Here's one thing about being over fifty: Exercise was invented after we were adults. I didn't grow up thinking "Of course I'm supposed to exercise." I grew up running around, bicycling, playing games, and being active just because I liked it. The good news is this: now that we've invented exercise, people start doing it earlier and are more likely to keep doing it.

In the real world, most people don't get to the gym as often as they'd like. Usually that's because a trip to the gym takes at least a couple of hours out of an already busy day (at least, that's what we tell ourselves). So here's the first thing I want to tell you: You don't need to spend hours a day in pursuit of fitness. In fact, most experts now agree that you can get health benefits from just thirty minutes of exercise a day, five days a week. Even better, if you can't commit to thirty minutes all at once, three ten-minute bursts will still do your body good.

Believe me, I'm not saying you should stop going to the gym or taking your morning run. I'm just saying that it's better to do whatever you can whenever you can than to do nothing at all. It's better to make exercise a regular part of your lifestyle than to join a gym, do strenuous workouts for a month, and then stop going. The most important thing is to keep moving—especially as you get older, and especially if you are a woman. We all lose muscle as we age (starting from around age thirty), but in women, loss of muscle mass increases sixfold at the time of menopause. That's one reason strength training is so important for women in their fifties and beyond.

If you do go to the gym, consider working with a personal trainer at least some of the time. A trainer can help you determine what exercises are best for you, show you how to develop a routine, let you know when you're doing something wrong, pat you on the back when you're making progress, and motivate you to keep moving.

Notes from Oscar Smith

As you get older, you become more susceptible to injuries and it takes longer to recover, so you've got to be careful not to overexercise, especially if you haven't worked out in a while. That's not to say you can't build up your fitness capabilities at any age; you can, and you should. But you have to work out differently than you did when you were younger. Diversity is key, because you want to cover all the major muscle groups. Change your workout every few days—run, swim, ride a bike. Use a variety of machines at the gym. Don't just hit the treadmill; switch off to the elliptical machine. Start slowly and build up your endurance. The idea is not to exhaust yourself but to challenge your body.

It's not helpful to compare yourself with the way you looked when you were younger. You may not be able to get back to that weight or shape. But you can be more fit and attractive for your current age, and feel better as well, if you exercise regularly.

When choosing a gym, make sure it is adequate for your needs. Does it have enough machines to keep you challenged? Does it offer a variety of classes—not just aerobics, but perhaps yoga or Pilates as well? Check out the atmosphere. You don't necessarily want to go where bodybuilders and professional athletes train, but be sure that the staff and trainers are knowledgeable and helpful. And find a gym that's close to home or work. The longer it takes you to travel there, the less often you'll go.

It's good to work with a personal trainer at the gym. A trainer can help you in many ways, initially by giving you a fitness assessment to tell you where your strengths and weaknesses lie and what areas need the most attention. Then he or she can teach you various exercises and routines, show you proper form, and help you apply that knowledge to new exercises as you progress. You don't need a trainer if you're only using the machines, as most machines have little instruction charts on them. You should use a trainer when you need to be challenged and you're ready to step up your exercise program to the next level. A trainer will push you further than you might go by yourself.

My best piece of exercise advice is this: *Don't get discouraged.* As with everything else in life, progress in baby steps. Stick with it, and you'll improve your health and look great at the same time.

Notes from David Barton

Exercise really is the fountain of youth. The tangible effects of aging are the result of a breakdown of tissue in the body, particularly protein tissue, for which there is one antidote: lifting weights. Strength training restores protein metabolism as well as muscle and bone density, and it reinvigorates every organ of the body. I'm not just talking about aging gracefully; I'm talking about turning a fifty-year-old body into a youthful, dynamic, beautiful, thirty-five-year-oldish body. If you're over the age of thirty-five, every year you lose about half a pound of muscle (which slows the metabolism) and gain about a pound and a half of body fat. In ten years you've lost five pounds of muscle, but you're ten pounds heavier. Do the math—that's ten pounds every decade. So you become fatter, softer, and weaker. And as you continue to lose lean muscle tissue, your metabolism gets even slower, and you are set up for continual weight gain.

The only scientifically proven solution to this muscular deterioration and weight gain is lifting that dumbbell. The best thing to do is go to a gym and begin to work with a trainer, an expert who will teach you how to pump iron the right way. Every day, I see people in my gym who are slowing their aging processes. I recently saw a woman who appeared to be in her forties; it turned out she was sixty-nine. Other people her age already look and act very old. Being active and lifting those weights make all the difference. Exercise not only helps you to stay healthy and mobile but also gives you the opportunity to lead as dynamic and interesting a life as anyone at any age.

77

Notes from Suzanne Meth

Exercise should be a regular part of our lives for many reasons. It strengthens the body and empowers us in other areas of our lives. People who exercise on a regular basis are more confident, both physically and mentally. They have sharper minds and are better decision-makers.

But exercise is even more important for women once they reach forty and perimenopause. Their metabolism slows down, their energy decreases, and they start to experience hormonal changes, mood swings, hot flashes, and a loss of estrogen. The loss of estrogen is one reason women put on weight and have difficulty losing those pounds as they age. A study by Dr. Andrew Greenberg of Tufts University published in the *Journal of Biological Chemistry* (October 2005) stated, "When estrogen was present in muscle, liver, and fat cells, the expression of genes that control manufacturing and storing fat was reduced, and the expression of genes that promote burning fat in muscle cells was in-creased." In other words, when we have more estrogen, we store less fat and burn more of it as well. So when estrogen naturally drops, the body hoards fat to make up for the loss. The more estrogen we lose, the more reluctant the body is to give up fat cells. There are certain things we can't fight. We can certainly work to get fitter and leaner, but it's better for our mental health to accept that some additional weight is part of getting older.

It's unfortunate that our society is so youth oriented. Women are expected to maintain their youthful looks no matter what their age, as if looking twenty were the norm. I encourage people to have realistic goals. People often give up on exercise because they set goals they can't reach overnight. If their expectations are too high and unrealistic, they're never going to look the way they think they should.

Youthfulness is largely a state of mind and a question of switching to a positive mind-set. Why do you have to focus on your love handles? No one else does. It's important to realize that there is no universally ideal body. Fitness is a continuum. You never arrive there. There's never a day when you can say, "I'm done. I'm good. I can stop now." It's much healthier to begin an exercise program by focusing on how much more you can do and how much better you will feel than you did before you started.

The Body Age Test

One of the services available at the Equinox Club is the Polar BodyAge machine, which gauges one's body age compared with one's chronological age. Through a series of measurements (ranging from eating habits to medical conditions, family history, and risk factors for various diseases) and physical tests (measuring body composition, heart fitness, muscular strength, flexibility, height, and weight), we are able to determine how much "younger" or "older" a body is than the actual number of biological years it has aged. For instance, although you may be chronologically thirty-five years old, our tests may show that because of your poor eating habits, family history of diabetes, and lack of flexibility, your "body age" is closer to fifty.

We measure your fuel utilization, which is how well you use fats and carbohydrates, and your VO_2, which stands for volume of oxygen consumed, or how efficient your body is at delivering oxygen to your muscles. We take your medical history to determine your risk for skin cancer (almost everyone rates high on this risk), breast cancer, colon cancer, and diabetes—diseases that can run in families. We also take a "state-trait anxiety inventory," a test that measures degrees of stress and anxiety. And we use calipers to measure your body composition. Lean body mass is made up of water, bone, muscles, and organs—everything but fat.

In the case of Irja, a fifty-five-year-old woman, the body age test showed her real body age to be sixty-three. Taking everything into account—including her family history, which she cannot change—if she eats right and trains properly, she should be able to get her body age down to thirty-five. That would be her goal. The body age test made the following recommendations:

- Improving skin cancer health risk from "potential" to "low" would improve her body age by five years.

A GOOD MOTIVATOR

Oz suggested I take the body age test because I was having trouble losing weight and wasn't sure why. I used to go to the gym years ago and work with a trainer. But in the past ten years, I haven't gone at all. So I think the test results are quite useful as a guideline and as a motivator to get you going again.

It's a little skewed because it's multiple choice, so it doesn't take different circumstances into consideration. I live in England, and the protocols for certain cancer screenings are slightly different from the protocols in the United States. The protocol for mammograms, for instance, is every second year here (as opposed to every year in America). So that put me in the category of risk for breast cancer. Also, they did a nutritional analysis, asking about the foods I eat. Some of that was difficult for me, too, because we don't have the same things in the supermarket here. We don't eat the same foods, apart from general things like getting enough fiber and fresh fruits and vegetables and drinking water.

The most important piece of information for me was realizing I need to do more cardiovascular work. That came from the test where you breathe and they measure how much oxygen you use—your resting and working metabolism. Since I took the test I've been traveling like crazy and crazy busy, so I haven't yet had an opportunity to improve. But I do plan to go back to the gym and work with a trainer.

I tested "mild" on the stress level meter. That's because I have a stress-free life. I paint and I do yoga; this is what I spend my time doing. Hence the low blood pressure. My children are grown up and they've moved on, and that's also why I have such low blood pressure. But other tests were higher, such as for colon cancer, because I have a family history in that area.

I think the test is excellent if you're working with somebody like Oz, or with a personal trainer, so they will be more informed about your particular circumstances. They can use the results for motivation and for showing you what you need to do; this is what's lacking and that's where you're falling behind, and so on. Then it's really useful.

If someone is age forty and they test at age seventy-five, this test may be what they need to set them on a healthier course. My real body age did take me by surprise, even though it's not so many years off. I'm fifty-five, and my body age came out to be sixty-three. They tell me that if I work really hard, I can get my body age down to around thirty-five.

IRJA BRANT, FIFTY-FIVE,
MOTHER OF TWO

- Improving colon cancer health risk from "severe" to "low" would improve her body age by five years.
- Improving diabetes health risk from "high" to "low" would improve her body age by five years.
- Improving stress health risk from "mild" to "low" would improve her body age by three years.
- Improving body composition from 28.6 percent to 21.09 percent would improve her body age by five years.
- Improving cardiovascular VO_2 score from 24 to 31.9 would improve her body age by three years.

Of course, these results were particular to Irja, her situation, her health concerns, and her family background. Everyone who takes the test comes up with a personalized result. Some people score very close to their chronological ages, while others score further away. Whatever the results, the test indicates that making even small changes in your lifestyle, diet, and exercise habits can add years to your life.

81

Oz Wraps It Up

Irja's results are not unusual for a woman, nor would it be unusual for a man to test at a higher body age. Granted, a lucky few are able to coast late into life with minimal support. For instance, some people are genetically endowed to have better muscle mass whether or not they work out. Others can cope with a significant amount of stress whether or not they're taking time off, getting massages, or sleeping eight hours each night.

The majority of us, however, require a lot of upkeep as we get older. The simple fact of aging calls for more intensive personal maintenance. We could get away with a great deal more when we were younger, but as we get older we can no longer take our health and physical abilities for granted.

The body age test will reflect the results of your lifestyle history. Perhaps you drink too much alcohol. Perhaps you skip meals. Perhaps you overextend yourself in any number of ways. The point is that it will all catch up with you. The good news is that no matter what your body age may be today, you can take immediate steps—no matter how small—to start reclaiming the years that hard living and certain lifestyle choices have taken away.

PART III

BEAUTY:

FACING UP TO AGING

"Nature gives you the face you have at twenty;
it is up to you to merit the face you have at fifty."

—COCO CHANEL

HOW DO YOU define beauty? The Merriam-Webster Online Dictionary defines it as "the quality or qualities in a person or thing that gives pleasure to the senses or pleasurably exalts the mind or spirit." Wikipedia (a free online encyclopedia with entries that are continuously being edited and updated by contributors around the world) defines it as "an innate and emotional perception of life's affirmative aspects—vitality, health, fertility, happiness, and goodness—within objects in the *perceived world*. In its most profound sense, beauty engenders a sense of positive reflection on the meaning of one's own being within nature."

Unfortunately, we are not always so lofty when defining beauty—especially as it refers to aging. We live in a youth-oriented, Hollywood-obsessed society where women often get "extreme makeovers" in pursuit of beauty and often end up looking like cartoon characters with exaggerated duck lips on faces that have no ability to show expression, and breast implants larger than the state of Rhode Island.

In *Redesigning 50* we have a whole new approach to beauty and how we look while we're aging. There are many new, exciting, non–plastic-surgery technologies that can help women age beautifully without trying—and inevitably failing—to make them look twenty years old. Going under the knife is always a choice, and we talk a little bit about it in chapter 7, but it is not for everyone. I believe it should be considered only as a last-resort option. I always tell my clients who are considering plastic surgery to make some lifestyle changes first and see what happens—follow the New 50 Fusion Food Plan, exercise, get plenty of rest, see a dermatologist, and learn to take care of your skin. If you can do those things, you probably won't need plastic surgery after all.

NOT FOR WOMEN ONLY

The fact that women's skin is more sensitive than men's doesn't mean that men don't have skin problems, too. Men show the same signs of aging as women—wrinkles, age spots, and so forth—although they may appear later than they do for women. Some men never even think of skin care or dismiss it as something that is just for women. But men can take steps to improve their appearance, too. Here are a few easy tips to keep a man's skin looking young and healthy:

- *Get a Facial:* Find a spa that caters to both men and women. Even if you get only one facial in your life, it can be very helpful to have a professional esthetician tell you about your skin type and educate you about various techniques and products that will best suit your needs.
- *Get a Professional Shave:* For the same reason you should get a facial, have a pro give you hints and techniques and recommend products that will give you the best shave and keep your skin healthy at the same time.

■ *Avoid Alcohol-Based Aftershaves:* The alcohol will irritate your skin. Find a soothing gel or moisturizer instead.

■ *Avoid Excess:* Smoking, alcohol, stress, and fatigue will accelerate the aging of your skin. Alcohol is particularly dehydrating, which is why you look sallow the morning after a night of drinking.

■ *Use Cosmeceuticals Designed for Men's Skin:* Cosmeceuticals are topically applied products that deliver nutrients and contain ingredients that influence the biological function of the skin. Among them are cleansing products that don't contain commercial dyes and fragrances that can irritate the skin and clog pores.

■ *Keep Up the Exercise:* Exercise increases the amount of oxygen that reaches skin tissue and keeps the skin looking young and vibrant.

■ *Be Vigilant about Skin Cancer:* Both men and women are more prone to skin cancer as they age. Wear sunscreen as often as possible, even on cloudy days, and don't forget your face, your ears, the back of your neck, and any bald spots. Wear sunglasses to protect your eyes, as sun exposure increases your risk of getting cataracts. And visit a dermatologist to have a body check for any signs of skin cancer. You can do a preliminary check of moles yourself, following the ABCDE rule to look for anything suspicious:

  • A—Asymmetry (one side of the mole looks different than the other)
  • B—Border (the edges of the mole are blurry or jagged)
  • C—Color (the mole is irregularly colored or has changed color recently, gotten lighter or darker, or appears blue, red, white, pink, purple, or gray)
  • D—Diameter (the mole is larger than a quarter inch in diameter)
  • E—Elevation (the mole is raised above the skin and has a rough surface)

Beauty *Is* Skin Deep

The skin is the body's largest organ, one that science is discovering more about every day. The outer layer, or epidermis, helps hold in moisture while it keeps unwanted water out. It contains stem cells as well as pigment-producing melanocytes that help protect us against sun rays. The middle layer of skin, the dermis, contains collagen, which keeps skin firm (but which begins to break down as we age, causing the skin to wrinkle and sag as the years go by), as well as hormones, neural connections that run to the brain, and nerve endings that interface with our environment. The bottom layer of skin is subcutaneous fat, which contains larger blood vessels and nerves and acts as a layer of insulation to help our bodies stay warm and absorb shocks. The subcutaneous fat lies on the muscles and bones, to which the whole skin structure is attached by connective tissues.

As it turns out, the skin is much more important than we once imagined as a protective instrument for our immune system, as a messenger of information regarding our current state of health and well-being, and as a mirror that clearly reflects our emotional state. We now know, for instance, that the skin can activate an immune response and trigger inflammatory responses throughout the body. We know that the skin produces hormones and is flush with neurotransmitters.

We also now know that there are tangible differences between the skin of men and women. Women's skin is thinner and tends to be less oily than men's. Both these factors make women's skin more vulnerable to changes in climate and to the damaging effects of the sun. Women are also at higher risk for skin cancer after menopause. Young skin contains both estrogen and testosterone; testosterone helps keep skin oily, and estrogen increases collagen and moisture. When women lose estrogen, however, they lose some of its benefits; the result is drier skin, less collagen, and more wrinkling and sagging.

In the following chapters, we discuss how valuable skin is, not only in the way you look but how interconnected it is with your overall health and well-being. We introduce you to several experts who discuss the available cutting-edge technologies for skin repair and rejuvenation, as well the latest cosmeceuticals. You'll also discover how to maintain a more youthful appearance with a few little tricks of hair and makeup from several of the country's top stylists, so you can improve how you look and feel from the outside in as well as the inside out.

The object is to honor your age and stage in life, to resist the temptations of our youth-obsessed society, and to find both your inner your outer beauty no matter what your age.

SIX

SKIN DEEP

ENTERING THE NO-PLASTIC-SURGERY ZONE

IF PEOPLE COULD see us without our skin, would they know how old we are? Physicians or medical examiners might be able to make an educated guess, but for most of us, the skin is what gives away a person's age. And although we may suffer from the internal aches and pains that make getting older a daily annoyance, it's often the visible signs of aging that drive us really crazy.

Unfortunately, there are no magic pills or miracle creams that will make us look twenty years younger while we sleep. There are, however, many new products and treatments available to help reduce some of those fine lines, wrinkles, sags, and spots we wish we didn't see in the mirror every day.

Of course, looking younger starts with proper nutrition, exercise, sleep, and stress reduction. All those factors will naturally help us look healthier and more vibrant, which automatically translates into looking younger. When we're young, we have a healthy supply of growth factors, enzymes, and hormones to keep us looking firm and fit, but this supply diminishes as we age. Combine this fact with less sleep, more stress, and harmful lifestyle choices such as eating, drinking, smoking, and tanning too much, and we've got the perfect formula for accelerated aging.

What do all those unhealthy lifestyle choices actually do to us? What is going on beneath the surface of the skin? Three primary processes make us look (and feel) old: oxidation, inflammation, and glycation. First, oxidation occurs when oxygen interacts with organic tissue, thereby producing the unstable oxygen molecules known as free radicals. Free radicals start a tissue-damaging chain reaction in our bodies that results in "microscarring," which causes wrinkles. Then the second damaging process begins: inflammation, which causes damage at the cellular level. The third villain in this scenario, caused by the overconsumption of sugar, is glycation, which occurs when sugar molecules bind to collagen molecules and make them stiff and prone to discoloration, better known as age spots.

What can you do about all this? We spoke to three great authorities on the subject, all of whom offer their own unique and equally impressive theories and solutions: geneticist Daniel Davidson, chairman, CEO, and founder of M.D. Darwin Labs, who looks at the problem from a genetics standpoint; Dr. Nicholas Perricone, dermatologist and author of several best-selling books, including *The Wrinkle Cure* and *The Perricone Promise*, who is an expert on inflammation; and endocrinologist and renowned public-health expert Dr. José Lladós-Comenge, who focuses on hormones. We also spoke to Gordon Chiu, a naturopathic doctor and international beauty and skin consultant.

All four of these experts believe in treating the skin from the inside out with products that have been developed from an understanding of the biology of aging. The products recommended by each have been tested and found to produce extraordinary results. You can choose which one makes the most sense for you and find information about where to get each of their products in the resource guide at the end of book.

Notes from Daniel Davidson on DNA and the Skin

Who would have thought that the Human Genome Project would be relevant to skin care? Here's how the connection was made. I began my career in genetics and biotechnology and eventually built the largest privately held genetics testing company in the United States. In 1990, the Human Genome Project was undertaken, with the goal of identifying all the approximately twenty- to twenty-five thousand genes in human DNA in order to understand the body at the molecular and genetic level. For the first time ever, doctors and scientists got real insights into how the body is structured, why it functions the way it does, why diseases manifest themselves the way they do, and what changes or external influences could be created to best combat some of these problems.

It's like having an architectural blueprint of the human body. Imagine having a building and trying to fix a problem without really understanding the air conditioning and the electrical and plumbing systems. It would be a blind endeavor with little chance of success. But once you've got the architectural blueprint, you can start to make levelheaded, rational decisions about how to approach these issues. That's what we can do, now that the Human Genome Project has given us the blueprint of the human body.

What interested me most was how the "secrets of youth" within our DNA could be applied to "fixing" aging. So my research began. I read about an enzyme called photolyase ("fot-o-lie-ase"), which occurs naturally in certain organisms that are exposed to the sun. When ultraviolet-B radiation from the sun hits cells, it destroys that beautiful double helix, the twisted ladder that we all know as DNA. Once this damage is encoded in our cells, it is naturally replicated over and over again. To repair the DNA, cells use photolyase to initiate chemical reactions that actually reverse the damage. Remarkably, this enzyme harnesses the energy of the sun—the initial cause of the problem—to repair the DNA.

If you look back in history, milky white skin was a sign of wealth; it meant you never had to toil in the fields to make a living. In fact, the very rich were called blue-bloods because you could see the blue blood of their veins through their thin white skin. In the twentieth century, having a suntan became a sign of wealth; it meant you had time to lie out in the sun. When scientists found out how damaging the sun is, they developed products to protect us from the sun's rays.

As you get older you want to help prevent the body from getting overwhelmed, to provide as much of a protective mechanism as you can. The products that our scientists have developed at M.D. Darwin Labs are based on many amazing breakthroughs in biotechnology, and not only help provide that protection but actually reverse some of the damage that's already been done. This is a first step toward creating a whole profile of skin-care products that are truly beneficial to the skin instead of just covering it. A study published in the February 2000 issue of *Proceedings of the National Academy of Sciences* found that the "the topical application of exogenous photolyase to human skin . . . is an approach that is highly efficient in protecting human skin from the deleterious effects that result from the presence of UVB-induced damage." The study also shows that by reversing DNA damage, you actually increase immunoprotection of the skin.

The skin has a natural immune system that is broken down when it's bombarded with environmental insults like ultraviolet-B radiation, making the skin less capable of defending itself against pathogens and other environmental influences. Once you start chiseling away at the integrity of the skin, it's not only sun damage you have to worry about—you're at much greater risk of infection. By keeping your skin healthy, you have a considerably greater chance of warding off some of these environmental insults.

Notes from Dr. Nicholas Perricone
on Inflammation and the Skin

I've been studying and lecturing about inflammation since the late 1980s. In my opinion, inflammation mediates the whole spectrum of aging. Even if your skin is affected by overexposure to the sun, it is inflammation that causes the underlying damage. In fact, inflammation at the cellular level is the single most powerful cause of the signs of aging (not to mention its relationship to chronic diseases like arthritis, diabetes, Alzheimer's, cancer, and strokes).

How does this relate to our skin? Unfortunately, this chronic sub-clinical inflammation is also a significant contributor to wrinkled, sagging skin. To combat this inflammation we need to follow a three-tiered program, whose cornerstone is the anti-inflammatory diet. Foods that are anti-inflammatory are foods rich in antioxidants such as brightly colored fruits and vegetables, as well as nuts, seeds, beans, and other legumes, and are also low on the glycemic index, which means they will not raise blood sugar and insulin levels when ingested. Antioxidant nutritional supplements and topical antioxidants will also protect against the damage. We also need adequate high-quality protein, such as salmon, so that the cells can repair themselves (a lack of protein accelerates aging and is first apparent in the face). Salmon contains a powerful antioxidant, an anti-inflammatory carotenoid known as astaxanthin, which helps keep skin supple and radiant.

As we age, the level of natural neuropeptides, amino acids produced by the body, diminish. We can apply natural neuropeptides to our skin daily to retain a youthful appearance and slow the signs of premature aging. These neuropeptides dramatically improve the appearance of skin in terms of resilience, tone, and texture, while decreasing the appearance of fine lines and wrinkles. With continued use, they also minimize the appearance of skin discoloration, redness, and puffiness. When neuropeptides are combined with DMAE (a powerful neurotransmitter precursor that protects cell membranes against degradation), they help restore a well-hydrated, revived, contoured appearance to the eye area; reduce the appearance of fine lines and wrinkles; increase balance and moisture; reduce the appearance of papery, translucent skin; increase the appearance of skin tone and firmness; and decrease the appearance of puffiness and dark circles.

Notes from Gordon Chiu on Beauty and Life Extension

As a consultant for many skin-care lines, it is my job to optimize the ingredients and the formulation of a variety of products. In other words, I take the products and make them better.

The skin is the largest organ of the body, and it's the body's first and best defense mechanism. You don't want to put anything on your skin that's going to weaken that barrier. You should be as careful with what you put on your skin as with what you put in your mouth.

One of the best products I've worked with is LaVigne Organic Skin Care, which contains two very special ingredients: Himalayan crystal salt and tepezcohuite (pronounced "tep-ez-co-heety"). Himalayan crystal salt, imported from the mountains of Pakistan, contains eighty-four minerals and trace elements essential to health; it is the same ingredient that makes Oz Water so good for you. Tepezcohuite is a primary healing and regenerative agent derived from the bark of Mexico's "skin tree," used by the Mayans for more than ten centuries as an antiaging skin-care product. Modern-day research has revealed that vital components found in its complex chemical makeup actually repair and protect skin cells, giving it the amazing ability to heal a wide range of skin problems and to promote younger-looking, healthy skin.

Of course, skin care is made up of more than just the products you use. I believe that there are eleven steps to quality skin that you can take for beauty and life extension (living life in the healthiest way possible—and looking good while you're doing it).

1. *Reduce or Eliminate Stress:* Your psychological state is reflected in the way you look.

2. *Be Careful What You Eat:* Following a healthy, balanced diet that includes fish, lean meats, and lots of fruits and vegetables can make a huge difference in your skin's health and appearance.

3. *Be Particular about What You Drink:* Don't just drink eight glasses of water a day—drink eight glasses of the best water available (*e.g.,* Glaceau Vitamin Water, Voss Water from Norway, or Oz Water with Himalayan crystal salt).

4. *Get Quality Sleep:* This gives your body time to repair itself. And don't discount the importance of your sleeping surface. For example, sleeping on natural fibers is much better for your skin than sleeping on synthetics.

5. *Strengthen Your Repair Efficiency:* Do you bruise easily? If you get a cut, how quickly do you heal? Be sure you are feeding your body the proper nutrients, through diet and supplementation, to help your body repair itself.

6. *Increase Your Blood and Lymphatic Circulation:* Keep your blood cells healthy with antioxidants (see chapter 13), and maintain proper levels of blood pressure and cholesterol. (Tepezcohuite, in fact, has strong antioxidant properties.)

7. *Be Sure You're Getting Adequate Amounts of Vitamins and Minerals:* Take proper supplements for your skin and hair as well as for your overall health. Fill your diet with fresh foods in season.

8. *Wash Your Skin Carefully:* Use products without harsh detergents.

9. *Moisturize:* Moisturizing is a good idea, but don't overdo it (you don't want to clog your pores), and be sure to use sun protection.

10. *Protect Yourself from Germs, Viruses, Fungi, and Bacteria:* Choose organic foods that don't use pesticides, and products from animals that are not fed hormones or antibacterial agents.

11. *Strengthen Your Immune System:* The better your body's ability to fight off disease naturally, the less you'll have to rely on artificial pharmaceutical products that can be harmful to your health and looks.

96

Notes from Dr. José Lladós-Comenge on Hormones and the Skin

Whatever happens inside your body is reflected in your skin. Any lifestyle and food choices you make will affect your overall physical appearance because all the body's systems are connected. I approach aging and skin-care issues with an understanding of the connection between the endocrine, immune, and nervous systems and the skin. It is a fusion of science and sensuality. My goal is to help people extend what I refer to as their sensual skin span—giving skin many more years of health, vitality, and youthful allure.

All hormones affect your skin, some more than others. For women, the skin is particularly affected by estrogen, the hormone that is produced by the ovaries; cortisol, the hormone that is produced when you are under stress; insulin, the hormone that helps the cells take in glucose and convert it to energy; and the thyroid hormones, which regulate metabolism.

My goal is to help the skin work the way it did when the hormones were functioning properly. When you're young, you produce estrogen and progesterone every month. These hormones help the skin to moisturize and exfoliate properly. As you approach your late thirties your estrogen levels decrease, which means your skin does not exfoliate as well as it used to and begins to get dry. Cortisol also affects the way your skin produces moisture and exfoliates, which is why you have skin problems such as eczema and acne when you're under stress. If you experience both an increase of cortisol and a decrease of estrogen at the same time, you will definitely see the damage appear on the surface of the skin.

Keeping your skin moist is very important because moisture will prevent lines and wrinkles. Traditional products moisturize your skin by putting fatty acids on the skin's surface, creating a "protective" layer that prevents water from leaving the skin and keeps the moisture in. However, that clogs the pores and doesn't allow the skin to breathe properly. Look for products that help the cells produce their own natural moisture from the inside out without clogging the pores.

Another factor to take into consideration is exfoliation. As you get older the turnover of the cells diminishes. When you're in your twenties, your cells renew every month. But as you get older your skin may need two or three months to renew itself. Traditional skin care has treated this problem by using alpha-lipoic, glycolic, and Retin-A acids to remove dead skin cells. While this approach may make the skin youthful again, we have found that frequent

97

use of these acids exposes your immune system, which is also in your skin, to potential damage and premature aging. If you are constantly applying acid to your skin, over time you will age faster.

In the end, what you really want is sensual skin. Healthy skin is moist and soft to the touch, even if you have lines and wrinkles. As we age, all our senses decline. Our eyesight gets worse; our hearing gets worse. And our sense of touch gets worse; we actually lose feeling. By returning the skin to its youthful health, you can restore the sense of touch that you may have lost.

Oz Wraps It Up

With so many skin-care products available today, it can be difficult to determine which ones are the best for you. It may take some trial and error. Visit a dermatologist and find out what he or she recommends. Stay away from anything that promises to perform miracles or sounds too good to be true. Don't forget the most basic advice: practice healthy nutrition, avoid too much sun, and stop smoking (which causes irreversible premature facial wrinkling). We boomers may be getting older, but there's no reason we can't look damn good while we do it!

SEVEN

ALTERNATIVE OPTIONS

FROM DERMATOLOGY TO MESOTHERAPY

IT'S AMAZING WHAT science and technology have to offer us today in terms of improving how we look. Before the twentieth century, one's appearance was pretty much determined by one's genes and environment. Wrinkles, sags, scars, big noses, small lips—they were there for life, for better or for worse. We now live in a very different time, when improving on nature is as commonplace as upgrading our cable service.

That is not to say that in earlier times everyone had a *que sera, sera* ("what will be, will be") attitude about appearance. Throughout history, humankind has sought self-improvement. Tombs from the First Dynasty of Egypt (ca. 3100–2907 BC) were discovered to contain unguent jars. Unguent was a substance used extensively by men and women to keep their skin hydrated and supple and to avoid wrinkles from the dry heat. And historians have noted that primitive forms of medical treatment for facial injuries (what we now know as plastic surgery) were performed more than four thousand years ago.

Our twenty-first-century world offers a lot more than unguents and treatment for facial injuries. Between plastic surgery news articles and reality shows, you'd think that surgery was your only option to look younger. However, there are many less drastic, less invasive options, and this chapter discusses several of them. While this book is essentially a "no-plastic-surgery guide," many people are curious about it, so there is also some discussion of plastic surgery should you consider going that route.

The experts who have provided information on some of the available options are Dr. Lisa Zdinak, an ophthalmic plastic surgeon with specialty training in advanced techniques in minimally invasive facial rejuvenation; Dr. Lisa Airan, a cosmetic dermatologist and clinical instructor at Mt. Sinai Hospital; Dr. Z. Paul Lorenc, plastic surgeon, clinical professor of plastic surgery at New York University School of Medicine, and author of *A Little Work*; and Dr. Lionel Bissoon, president of the American Board of Mesotherapists and author of *The Cellulite Cure*.

Notes from Dr. Lisa Zdinak on Eyelid Surgery and Nonsurgical Skin Therapies

Whether you're considering "having some work done" or trying to find a nonsurgical route to improving your appearance, you have many options available to you. You can choose either to have one procedure done or a series of procedures for a total facial rejuvenation.

As an oculoplastic surgeon, the first thing I notice about a person is the eyes. Signs of aging often appear around the eye area with the drooping of the upper eyelids and bags and wrinkles under the eyes. I was trained specifically to perform cosmetic surgeries on the delicate eyelid structures, eyelids and fatty bags can be treated a variety of ways. Unlike many surgeons, when I operate on the eyelids I do not use a scalpel on those candidates who opt for surgery. Instead, I use a precision Ellman Surgitron Radiosurgical device that emits radiowaves to make precise incisions and to minimize recovery time and complications.

Surgery can be effective for many people, but it is not the only means to recapture the look of youth. In fact, the majority of my patients want to improve their appearance without the downtime associated with surgery. There

THE EYES HAVE IT

They say the eyes are the window to the soul, and I wanted my windows to look as young as I feel. A few years ago, I had the fat removed from underneath my eyelids in a procedure called blepharoplasty, which is used to correct "puffy bags" below the eyes and drooping upper lids that make some people look older and tired or that interfere with vision. A good eye surgeon goes in and just removes a decent amount of fat—but not too much, because as you get older you can actually get too hollow.

I also had a carbon dioxide laser treatment that resurfaces the skin on my upper and lower eyelids. It helped to smooth out the "crepey" look. The recovery was a little longer than I expected. There was a certain amount of redness that lasted a few months rather than a few weeks. But I was still pleased with the results.

I felt that my eyes were the one thing that gave away my age. I did before it became a huge problem. I felt that if I waited until I was in my mid-fifties to have it done, people would have said, "Oh, you got your eyes done." This way, it was so subtle even my mother didn't know I did it. You shouldn't look as if you've had eye surgery. For me, it was a wonderful thing to do in terms of building confidence and feeling good and looking younger. Now, most people think I'm in my thirties.

JOHN ASLANIAN, FIFTY-FOUR,
MEDICAL MANAGEMENT CONSULTANT

are many aspects of the face and body that need to be addressed for optimal anti-aging results. To achieve a more youthful appearance, I have designed a unique variety of non-invasive treatment combinations, using the most advanced technology and products available. I define this highly effective approach as the "Precision Aesthetics Non-Surgical Face Lift." For these patients I have designed a regimen of nonsurgical therapies using injectable treatments, including Botox and injectable fillers, lasers, light sources, and Thermage. The foundation of my nonsurgical approach to facial and body rejuvenation is Thermage, a procedure that produces an immediate tightening effect. Thermage, using radio-frequency energy to heat the collagen in the deeper layers of the skin while gently cooling and protecting the skin surface, can be performed on the eyelids, face, neck, abdomen, arms, and thighs.

THE DARK CIRCLE DILEMMA

One of the most visible signs of aging for many people is the dark circles that appear under the eye. One new treatment provided by Dr. Zdinak is carbon dioxide therapy, or carboxytherapy: the administration of minute amounts of carbon dioxide gas just beneath the skin surface. It is a relatively painless, in-office procedure that is completed in five minutes with no residual downtime.

Carbon dioxide is a natural constituent of our very being. We breathe in oxygen, and we exhale carbon dioxide. Plants take up the carbon dioxide and in turn give us the oxygen we need (hence the common claim that plants thrive when you talk to them). Carbon dioxide also happens to be the signal for poor blood circulation in the body. All cells in the body, regardless of their function (heart cells, brain cells, skin cells) release carbon dioxide as waste. Carbon dioxide is the "cost of doing business" of any cell in our bodies. So we breathe oxygen into our lungs, and the red blood cells pick up the oxygen and carry it to our tissues until they encounter an area that has been working hard and has an excess of carbon dioxide. When the red blood cells are exposed to high concentrations of carbon dioxide, they flip their conformation, release the oxygen molecules, and pick up the carbon dioxide so that we can exhale it from our lungs. In a sense, by injecting small amounts of carbon dioxide gas just below the surface of the skin, we are tricking red blood cells into increasing blood circulation to that area.

Carboxytherapy can dramatically improve the appearance of dark under-eye circles. Although these dark circles are sometimes the result of darkened pigment, or a hollow depression below the lower eyelids (known as tear trough deformity), most of them are caused by poor circulation beneath the lower eyelids (or vascular pooling). Dr. Zdinak designed and conducted the first study in English using carboxytherapy for rejuvenating the under-eye region. She found that by injecting a small amount of carbon dioxide gas just beneath the skin of the lower eyelid, circulation was increased and dark under-eye circles were markedly improved. The treatment takes only five minutes and is virtually painless and risk-free. A series of two to six treatments spaced one week apart is all that is required to achieve a great result that lasts for about six months.

When used in proper combination, these treatments not only postpone the need for surgery but actually improve the surgical result when the time comes for a procedure in the future.

Once a patient has taken care of the eyes, face, neck, and arms, he or she often says, "If only there was something you could do for my hands." Some people say a person's hands can give away his or her age. For a total hand rejuvenation, a combination therapy is used. I start therapy by using Thermage on their hands. Depending upon the amount of sun exposure, you might have some dark spots, or age spots. Some people actually have very prominent veins on the surface of their hands. I use Thermage for the dark spots, and I use Intense Pulse Light and chemical peel to conceal the veins. There's a filling agent called Sculptra, a powder that is reconstituted into sterile water, which can help conceal the veins in the hand.

Patients sometimes ask me when they should begin these kinds of procedures. I tell them the sooner the better, because the younger you are, the more baseline collagen you have and the better your results will be. If you're older, you also probably have had more exposure to the sun, simply because you've been on the planet longer.

Whether you are looking to go under the knife or not, the important thing to remember is that you have options. A doctor who is trained in both surgical and nonsurgical techniques has a greater ability to meet your needs using methods custom designed for you.

Notes from Dr. Lisa Airan on Laser Treatments

When people come to a cosmetic dermatologist, it's because they really don't want to have surgery. They know they want to look better, but they may not

103

know exactly what they want or need. I always hand them a mirror and ask, "What bothers you the most?" Most people have something that really bothers them, even if it's something nobody else ever notices. I always focus first on the area that most concerns the patient, unless there's something that's really noticeable to me—for instance, if a woman had silicone implanted in her lips earlier that has now, after several years, become misshapen. She might think that nothing can be done about it, and I'll point out how I can help restore the balance to her face. But that's the exception. Otherwise, I want to be her advocate and work on the area that most bothers her, because I want her to feel good about herself.

As people age, they begin to have issues with the quality of their skin. The signs of aging in the face—in the skin itself—are broken blood vessels, brown spots, and dyschromia, which is discoloration or uneven skin tones. The skin no longer has that gorgeous milky glow of youth, but is damaged and sun battered. There are many techniques I can use to help patients look better, including various noninvasive therapies.

For instance, there's Thermage, the radio frequency device for skin tightening. With each touch to the skin, the Thermage device uniformly heats a large volume of collagen in the deeper layers of the skin and its underlying tissue while simultaneously cooling and protecting the outer layer of the skin. This heating action causes deep structures in the skin to tighten immediately. Over time, new and remodeled collagen is produced to tighten the skin further, resulting in healthier, smoother skin and a more youthful appearance. It's an effective and noninvasive way to help stimulate the production of elastin and collagen in the skin to give patients tightening along the jawline, in the nasal labial folds, and along the brow. The results last anywhere from two to three years; however, some patients prefer to have yearly touch-ups.

Another less invasive method is Gentle Waves LED Photomodulation, a light-based therapy that produces light-emitting diodes rather than thermal energy. The Gentle Waves technology delivers natural wavelengths of light that stimulate the production of collagen, similar to the way that sunlight stimulates plant life. There is no pain, no discomfort, and no side effects. The benefits include smoother, healthier skin and a gradual reduction in the appearance of wrinkles, fine lines, age spots, redness, and minor scarring. Although you don't see any immediate change when you leave the office after the first treatment, you will see results over the course of treatment, which usually takes eight to twelve weeks. This treatment is a good substitute for patients who can't use topical retinoic acid (Retin-A), which can give you similar results.

Then there are Intense Pulsed Light devices (IPLs) that use light absorption, whereby the light is changed to heat energy as it reaches the level of collagen beneath the skin's surface. The effect it produces is known as photonic rejuvenation. These devices are used for evening out skin tone, removing brown spots, and reducing redness in the skin.

To eliminate broken blood vessels, I use a device called Lyra. With one or two treatments, I can get rid of the unsightly blood vessels on the face or body, which may be due to sun damage, smoking, heredity, hormones, or steroid therapy. The laser light penetrates the skin, keeping it intact until it reaches the targeted blood vessel, which is immediately absorbed. At this point, the energy turns into heat and destroys the target without harming any surrounding tissue. It then takes a short while for the hair or vessel to dissipate into the body. This treatment is used not only for blood vessels but also for age spots.

105

Notes from Dr. Z. Paul Lorenc on Botox, Fillers, and Plastic Surgery

Many things make you look older, including, of course, environmental factors such as sun exposure and smoking, and biological factors that produce thinner, less pliable, and dryer skin. But as we move into our thirties and forties, several things begin to happen to the structure of the skin.

I'll start from the top. The brow descends. We see the beginning of transverse lines in the forehead and in the glabella, the area between the eyebrows. These lines occur because of hyperactivity of the underlying muscles. Aging also promotes fullness of the upper eyelids, when the supratarsal folds begin to lose definition. As children, we don't have any bags, so to speak, around the eyes. And through our mid-thirties, we usually have a very well-defined indentation where the muscle that opens the upper eyelid is located. Later, that definition gets blunted, fat becomes more pronounced, and the skin is not as tight or pliable. Wrinkles appear, and the upper eyelids become "hooded."

In the midface, there is a structure called the malar fat pad that covers the malar bone, the prominent cheekbone. As we age, the malar fat pad descends and causes two things to happen. First, its descent accentuates the nasal labial folds, the wishbone-like folds that bracket the area from the sides of the nose to the outer corners of the mouth. A young face has only a slightly defined nasal labial fold. As the fat pads descend more rapidly in our forties and fifties these folds become more accentuated.

When you move into your fifties and sixties, the fat descends even more quickly, leaving an indentation between the eyelid and the malar fat pads (and dark circles under the eyes). As the malar fat pads continue to descend, they force the beginning of jowls as the skin surrounding the ligament attachments at the jawline becomes lax. In the neck, you'll see a combination of a loss of skin tone, a prominence of muscle bands, and fatty deposits. The skin's loss of elasticity and the pull of gravity over time create an awful lot of facial changes as the years go by.

Whether or not you should have plastic surgery is an individual decision. If it's important enough to you, and you want to do it, then you should. However, for people in their thirties and forties, we start off with less invasive, nonsurgical ways to rejuvenate the face. Wrinkles are caused in part by the repeated contraction of the muscles used in facial expressions (frowning, laughing, furrowing the forehead). Even in your early thirties, you can minimize the activity of the muscles by using Botox to reduce formation of the transverse lines or wrinkles on the upper third of the face. Botox blocks signals from the nerves to the muscles and lasts up to six months. Botox injections have become the most common nonsurgical procedure in this country: between three and five million procedures are performed annually.

Another nonsurgical rejuvenation option for the face is represented by fillers, materials that plump up an area, most commonly the nasal labial folds (the skin crease extending from the nose to the corner of the mouth). But we

A LITTLE BOTOX NOW
AND THEN

I've done Botox twice now. The last time I did it was two years ago, and then I did it again about a month ago. I don't seem to get that frozen look people always make fun of. I decided to do it because it seemed like a noninvasive way of turning back the clock a bit. I knew that even if I didn't like the result, it was going to wear off in time. It wasn't permanent. And I know a fair number of people who've had it done, and I saw their results, so it didn't seem like something that was "out of the norm."

I have these two frown lines right in between my eyebrows, so that's where I had the Botox injected, and then the doctor did a little around the eyes for the crows' feet. No one else could tell that I'd had anything done or even commented on it. I'm not one of those people who pass a mirror and look. I don't study myself. But this time, when I had it done I said, "I want to pay attention; let me look at myself beforehand so that I can see the difference." It wasn't huge, but it was just enough to make me feel better.

It's really not a big deal, just a few shots. Afterward you can't lie down for four hours or get horizontal for four hours. No working out. And you have to scrunch your face a lot so that it doesn't get frozen. So for four hours afterward, I scrunched my face and didn't get supine.

JAN HOERRNER, FIFTY-TWO, RAISES CAPITAL AND
HANDLES INVESTOR RELATIONS FOR A PRIVATE EQUITY FIRM; MOTHER OF TWO

can also inject fillers into the upper lip, the "marionette lines," which go from the corners of the mouth to the chin, and the lines between the eyebrows. Botox works better between the brows, but you can also use a filler and sometimes a combination of the two. Right now, ten to fifteen fillers are available. A good filler should be safe and approved by the U.S. Food and Drug Administration (FDA). Ideally, it should last from one to two years and be totally biocompatible.

I prefer to use hyaluronic acid, a sugar found in large amounts in the synovial fluid, a thick liquid that assists in lubrication and nutrition of the joints. It attracts and holds almost a hundred times its weight in water, so it's a good moisturizing magnet. One of the most popular fillers is Restylane, made of biodegradable hyaluronic acid. Restylane treatments typically last about six months. During that time, Restylane is gradually degraded by the body and dissolves without leaving any residue.

But fillers can only fill so much. When you need something more, you may want to consider plastic surgery. It is my job to help my patients decide when plastic surgery is appropriate. It is very important to give patients realistic expectations. If I get a sense that they're expecting an impossible result, I have to tell them that surgery is probably not a good idea. Unfortunately, a lot of what goes on in the media right now perpetuates these unrealistic expectations. It downplays the fact that aesthetic plastic surgery is real surgery with real risks and long recovery times. Consequently, it has become more difficult for surgeons to present the experience to patients in realistic terms.

My best advice is to remember that this is completely elective surgery, so elect to be smart about it. This is not an emergency. Take all the time you need to find the surgeon who has the right credentials and makes you feel confident that you are going to be in the right hands.

A NOTE ABOUT LIPOSUCTION

 The most common misconception about liposuction is that it's a way to lose weight. It is not. It's a contour-correction modality. First of all, the skin must have pliability and elasticity so that when the fat is removed, the skin contracts without leaving ripples or indentations. A patient who is morbidly overweight or who has lost so much weight that the skin has lost its elasticity may make the situation worse by getting liposuction. For most patients, no more than six or seven pounds of fat are removed; otherwise, there may be serious health risks.

A good candidate for liposuction is someone who exercises on a regular basis and has a relatively good diet.

Notes from Dr. Lionel Bissoon on Mesotherapy

Mesotherapy, although a staple in Europe for more than forty years, is relatively new to this country. A mesotherapy practitioner injects microscopic quantities of natural extracts, homeopathic agents, pharmaceuticals, and vitamins into the skin to treat a variety of conditions. These tiny amounts of medication, which are highly specific to the condition being treated, are delivered directly to the mesoderm (the middle layer of the skin).

Mesotherapy can be used to treat everything from migraine headaches to back pain, malfunctioning metabolism, problems with the immune system, and health-related issues ranging from insomnia to cigarette smoking. For example, you can use mesotherapy to control pain and inflammation, especially as you're getting older. Let's say you are taking a nonsteroidal medication, such as the over-the-counter product ibuprofen, for your back pain. This is going to have a generalized effect within the body and *may* eventually find its way to the site of the pain. With mesotherapy, we know exactly where the pain is located and where to inject the pain relief. Since the dose of the pharmacological agent is minuscule, the possibility of side effects is greatly reduced.

In America, mesotherapy has become very popular among women for treating cellulite and for weight loss. There are several reasons women get cellulite and men usually don't. First, women carry three different layers of fat in the buttocks, the saddlebags, and around the knees, and one layer of fat almost everywhere else. Men have only one layer of fat throughout their bodies. Biologically, the extra fat in women is there for storage, to be used in pregnancy and during times of famine. Also, women have generally thinner skin and weaker connective tissue than men. In men, the connective tissue is cross-linked like a chain-link fence; in women, it's like spokes, but the fibers are not crossed.

Cellulite is a disease of decreased circulation, decreased oxygen, and decreased nutrition. It's also a reflection of changes in hormones, specifically estrogen. Estrogen has significant effects on smoothing, relaxing, and opening the

109

blood vessels, thereby increasing blood flow and reducing pressure. When there is a decrease in estrogen, the blood vessels become weak and flabby and begin to lose their tone; delivery of oxygen and nutrients to the cells becomes impaired, and fluid can get trapped within the fat cells. Owing to the lack of oxygen and nutrition, the collagen fibers around the fat become weak and cannot be repaired. So the fat cells become inflamed, push out through the weakened fences of connective tissues, and cause the lumpy, bumpy appearance many women know and hate.

In mesotherapy, we inject the treatment directly into the site of the cellulite to repair the collagen, shrink the fat cells, and increase circulation. In effect, we're mending the fence.

I want to point out that nutrition and exercise are important parts of these results. Exercise doesn't get rid of cellulite because it only shrinks the fat cells; you still have to address the problems with the connective tissue and circulation. If you maintain a sensible diet and a sensible exercise program before the onset of cellulite, you will be in the prevention phase. By the time you come and see me, you're in the intervention phase. It's not a quick fix. If you come to me for weight loss, I will agree to do mesotherapy for weight loss only if you agree to change your eating habits and start on an exercise program.

A WORD OF CAUTION

It's important to remember that there are no quick fixes. Every doctor we spoke to stated that, in order for their procedures to be truly beneficial, patients need to remember the role of proper nutrition and exercise in looking younger and staying healthier. And no matter what you do, there are liabilities. If you work out too hard, even with the best trainer, it's always possible that you'll get hurt. If you eat the best foods, it's always possible that you'll be allergic to something that's healthy for almost everyone else. So it is with any type of beautification treatment: It is possible to have a negative reaction. Some people who have had Botox treatments complain of headaches. If you have had Restylane injected and have an extremely sensitive immune system, you may experience short-term redness and swelling. Everything comes with a "buyer beware" warning.

The skin is an organ, so anything you put on it or in it will have some effect in terms of how you feel. We now know that there are neuropeptides that can affect your skin and transmit information to your brain. Think of yourself as one complete, holistic entity: What takes place in one part of you is going to affect what takes place in another part. Once you understand that, you can make intelligent decisions about your skin care and maintenance, and you will enjoy a healthier, more youthful, and vibrant appearance for many years to come.

Oz Wraps It Up

There are many decisions to be made when it comes to improving your appearance, not only about which procedures you want, but about who you want to perform them. In today's option-filled world, you can choose to go to several different doctors for different procedures, but it is important to note that nonsurgical procedures such as laser skin treatments, filling agents, or Botox injections may be performed by a dermatologist, plastic surgeon, cosmetic surgeon, facial plastic surgeon, or oculoplastic plastic surgeon.

Choosing a new physician may seem like an intimidating process, but there are ways that you can find the right match:

- *Choose a physician who underwent the proper training to address your specific problem.* There are many doctors who have extended the scope of their practice into the cosmetic realm as a means to enhance their incomes and to avoid dealing with medical insurance reimbursements. It is not unusual to hear about foot doctors giving Botox injections to the forehead, dentists doing facelifts, skin doctors doing eyelid surgery, and eye doctors doing breast implants! When seeking a practitioner for a cosmetic procedure, choose a surgeon who is committed to perfecting his or her technique through a residency and fellowship training program focused on the reconstructive and cosmetic procedures within the scope of that discipline. Physicians are not created equal. Dermatologists are medical doctors trained in the diagnosis and treatment of diseases of the skin. Some dermatologists have had several fellowships in microsurgical removal of skin cancers (MOHS procedure) and in hair transplantation. Plastic surgeons have the most comprehensive training in reconstructive and cosmetic procedures of the face and body. Be aware that a cosmetic surgeon does not undergo the same training as a plastic surgeon. A plastic surgeon has a minimum of five to seven years of required training, versus the minimum one year of required surgical training for a cosmetic surgeon.

■ *Don't pick a surgeon based on an advertisement.* Ask your current physician for the names of a few surgeons who he or she recommends. If you don't have a physician who can guide you toward someone they know personally, investigate the nearest academic hospital in your area (one that trains physicians) and seek out a surgeon with a teaching appointment in the discipline that you require. In order to teach residents, these individuals must have the highest credentials, including board certification and membership to fellowship societies. If you have a friend who is openly enthusiastic about his or her choice of physician, this can be the best recommendation of all. Only truly gifted physicians can establish a practice based primarily on referrals from existing patients. Once you have the names of at least three prospective surgeons, schedule a consultation visit with each one to see if you get along well.

Although your surgeon may be a skilled technician, he or she must respect your preferences. You should never feel as if the doctor is trying to "sell" you on something. If the physician is trying to persuade you to undergo a procedure, thank him or her for their time and then leave.

There is nothing wrong with wanting to look better or younger. It makes you feel good and bolsters your confidence. Perhaps most important, it can reflect the way you feel inside. As long as you don't get caught up in an elusive search for perfection or believe that your outward appearance is more important than who you are, why not take advantage of the many choices now available to help you look your best?

113

EIGHT

YOUR CROWNING GLORY

COMPONENTS OF BEAUTY FROM THE OUTSIDE IN

SAY WHAT YOU might about beauty being only skin deep—the fact is we all want to look good. There's something inexplicable about having your hair cut and colored by people who are truly artists at work, such as world-renowned stylist Edward Tricomi (affectionately known as Edward Scissorhands) and his salon partner, colorist Joel Warren, or by Frédéric Fekkai, one of the most celebrated names in beauty and hairstyling. And nothing makes you feel more glamorous than having someone do your makeup for you—especially someone like Bruce Dean, a makeup artist to stars such as Bette Midler, Kim Cattrall, and Linda Evangelista. And if you've ever dreamed of having the kind of smile that lights up a room, there's a new and exciting technique for making you and your teeth look ten years younger, as explained below by cosmetic dentist Dr. Marc Lowenberg.

Notes from Edward Tricomi on Hair

My generation was about burning bras, rock and roll, and pushing it forward. Now my generation is getting older, but we don't want to look like our mothers and fathers. Fortunately, we have developed a lot of styling tricks.

One trick is growing your hair longer to make you look younger—which is the opposite of what people usually tell you. But it's really a case-by-case decision. As a stylist, I look at a person's face, body, mentality, and manner of dress. I try to create a hairstyle to accommodate all that, but I also try to give my clients a little something extra. I can make them look their best at that point in time.

As an "older" woman you don't want to look like a teenager, but if you dress in a young, hip way and don't act old, you won't be old. There's also something to be said for growing old gracefully. When you come to a certain age, you can look really good and still be age-appropriate. It's all about having balance.

Another trick is hair coloring. One of the first things you notice as you get older is that your hair starts turning gray. Although there are some people who look great with gray hair, most people could use a little color to help them look and feel younger.

Notes from Joel Warren on Hair Color

You should color your hair in an age-appropriate way. If you're going to emulate someone's hair color, try to find someone who is within ten years of your age. And when you choose a hair color, don't stray too far from the natural color you had when you were young. If your hair was light brown, stay within two or three shades lighter or darker. If you were blond, stay blond; if you were dark brown, stay brown. Don't try to make a drastic change just because you reach a certain age.

The good news about hair coloring is that companies now make color that deposits moisture and protein in the hair and strengthens it, actually leaving your hair in better condition than before. People think that coloring your hair dries it out or damages it. The opposite is true as long as you keep coloring the regrowth when it comes in. When you start recoloring the ends, that's when you run into problems.

WHY DOES HAIR TURN GRAY?

Every strand of hair is made up of two parts: the shaft, which is the part we see, and the root, which keeps the strand anchored under the skin. The root is surrounded by a follicle sac, which contains blood vessels and hormone receptors, along with a certain number of pigment cells. Each follicle normally goes through a five-year cycle of growth and rest; about 90 percent of the follicles grow hair at any one time, averaging about six inches of growth per year. The pigment cells in the follicle produce melanin, which gives the shaft of the hair its color.

As we get older these pigment cells gradually die. With fewer pigment cells, the strand will contain less melanin and become more transparent as it grows. As this process continues we get grayer and grayer until eventually our hair is completely gray.

In terms of hair care, we're more fortunate than our parents' generation, because today we have the best skin and hair products in the world, formulated by the top scientists. There are hundreds of brands of products that work very well. One of the best products available is hair strengthener, which you use between shampooing and conditioning. Our brand is called Pure Strength. Conditioner is sort of like fabric softener—it makes your hair feel good—whereas strengthener actually restores and reinforces the hair, preventing it from breaking and splitting. But it all starts with having a great haircut.

Also, use highlights to give the hair definition, so it doesn't look like one solid color. Years ago, hair color was always monotone. It covered the gray, but it made you look older than it should have. Now you're able to incorporate other tones into your hair, which gives you more movement and a more natural look.

If you're coloring your hair at home, you've got to decide what type of product you need. The most important rule of thumb is that if you have more than 30 percent gray hair, you need a permanent hair color. If you have less than that, you can use a semipermanent or temporary color that will blend in the gray. Generally, women over fifty need a permanent hair color. When choosing that permanent hair color, try to stay close to your natural color, then play around with different shades of that color until you find the one that suits you best, and incorporate some highlights.

To take care of colored hair, I recommend using a strengthener. The hair cuticles overlap like shingles, forming the outermost layer of the hair shaft. When healthy and lying flat, these cuticles impart sheen to the hair. Over time, the hair cuticles open. When the cuticles open, the hair weakens, gets split ends, and looks dull. That's when you should use a strengthener. The difference between a conditioner and a strengthener is like the difference between a Band-Aid and an antibiotic—one covers the problem, and the other fixes it. A conditioner will help you manage your hair. A strengthener will help close down the cuticles of your hair, which will help strengthen it and restore some of the sheen that aging has taken away.

117

Words of Wisdom from Frédéric Fekkai

Caring for Your Hair: As you get older you have to be more careful about the way you care for your hair. Hydrate your hair with great treatments and conditioners. Be sure to rinse your hair well in the shower—never leave any residue on your hair unless you use a "leave-in" conditioner made specifically for that purpose.

Washing Your Hair: Wash your hair every day if you have fine, oily hair. Wash it every other day if you have thick, dry hair.

Using Conditioner: Here's a good tip that most people don't know: You don't need to condition the scalp. When working the conditioner into your hair, stay about an inch off the scalp, then comb the conditioner through and rinse it well.

Coloring Your Hair: Try not to make your hair very light or very dark. Those are shades you have when you are younger. As you age, your skin tone changes, so your hair should change as well. Everything should be organic. The more organic the coloring, the closer it is to your natural skin tone, the better you achieve a beautiful look. It's also important that the color have contrast so that it catches the light. If it's too flat, it looks like a cabinet.

Style: The length of your hair should vary with your height and the proportion of your body, not with your age. If you're long and tall, you can have longer hair, past the shoulder. If you're shorter, you're better off with hair that's shoulder length or shorter. If you have a rounder face, avoid bangs that go straight down your forehead; your bangs should be longer and swept to the side to counteract that round shape. If you have a longer, oval shape, try short bangs.

Finding a Good Stylist: When you see somebody with a great hairstyle—whether it's on the street, at the movies, or anywhere—ask that person who did her or his hair. Ask very fashion-conscious and style-conscious people for recommendations. Go into high-end stores such as Gucci and Chanel and ask the people who work there for the name of a good stylist or makeup artist. If you're not near one of those stores, go to a department store. Those people are usually plugged in.

Women over Forty: It's important that women over forty not try too hard. It's all in the editing. Don't put on too much makeup. Don't wear too much lipstick and lip liner. Don't overprocess your hair. Don't grow your nails too long. Don't put on too many accessories. You can have fun with your looks as long as you don't try to look as if you're twenty. With proper editing you can look youthful without trying to look young.

Getting to the Root of the Problem

One fact that men and women share is that we all lose hair as we age. According to the American Academy of Dermatology, the average human head has a total of ninety thousand to one hundred forty thousand hairs. Healthy heads lose fifty to one hundred hairs every day. As we age, that number increases. By the age of fifty, most of us have half the number of hairs we had when we were teenagers. The quality of the hair also changes. It becomes thinner, sparser, and grayer.

Unfortunately, many of us experience more hair loss than we'd like. There are several reasons:

Stress: Any kind of stress can contribute to hair loss—psychological trauma, illness, major surgery. That's one more good reason to find ways to manage the stress in your life. Usually, the hair loss isn't immediately noticeable; it may take up to three or four months before you notice the difference.

Hormonal Problems: People who have thyroid problems—both overactive and underactive—may experience hair loss as a side effect. Treatment of the disease can help in this instance. Other male and female hormones, known as androgens and estrogens, can cause hair loss when they are out of balance. When this imbalance is corrected, the hair loss will usually cease.

Medication: Everyone knows that chemotherapy usually causes hair loss, but so do some blood thinners (anticoagulants); antidepressants; certain medications for gout, arthritis, high blood pressure, and high cholesterol; and high doses of vitamin A. In some cases, the only way to stop the hair loss is to stop the medication; obviously, this is not something to do without consulting your health-care professional.

119

Nutritional Imbalances: A lack of protein, insufficient iron intake, and eating disorders can all take a toll on the health of your hair. Following the New 50 Fusion Food Plan can help, as can taking the supplements recommended in chapter 13.

Disease: Some illnesses, including lupus and diabetes, can cause hair loss. If you experience hair loss you can't explain, it's best to let your doctor know.

While women often experience thinning hair, men are more prone to alopecia, more commonly known as male pattern baldness. We all know the drill—the hairline gradually recedes and forms an M shape. The hair at the crown (the top of the head) starts to thin, creating a bald spot that gets larger and larger as time goes by. Eventually, the receding hairline meets the thinning crown, and all that's left is a fringe of hair around the sides of the head.

No one is really sure why this happens. Every hair on the head grows out of a cavity in the skin called a follicle. In men, the follicle shrinks over time, until only a tiny follicle remains with no hair inside it. Although there is no known way to stop this from happening, here are a few common treatment options:

Minoxidil: Sold under the brand name Rogaine, this medication is available without prescription and can be used by both men and women. It is rubbed directly onto the scalp to stimulate the hair follicle and thereby slow or prevent hair loss. In some people, it even promotes new hair growth.

Finasteride: Sold under the brand name Propecia, this medication is available by prescription only and is only for men. It is taken in pill form and works by inhibiting the production of the male hormone dihydrotestosterone. Hair loss returns when the person stops taking either minoxidil or finasteride.

Hair Transplants: This is accomplished by removing hair follicles from a different part of the body and grafting them onto the area of balding or thinning. There are minor risks of scarring or infection, and the procedure can be expensive. However, when the procedure is done by a highly qualified professional, the results are permanent, and no one can tell the difference (as opposed to many hairpieces, which can be spotted from a mile away).

Revita Shampoo: Revita is the most efficient hair growth-stimulating shampoo available in the market and is the final result of DS Laboratories' efforts on cutting-edge research. Revita is a powerful combination of precious materials specially designed to maintain scalp vitality and act on follicle dysfunctions in order to achieve best results in short periods of time. This formulation has been developed completely without the use of sodium lauryl sulfate and sodium laureth sulfate, commonly used low-cost detergents in shampoos and cleansers that are linked to skin irritation, drying, and hair loss due to follicle attack.

Spectral DNC Hair Treatment: Spectral DNC is a new medication that incorporates aminexil, a new, breakthrough compound that is the only other molecule aside from minoxidil that has been clinically proved to regrow hair. Other active ingredients include research-grade minoxidil 5 percent, adenosine, procyanidin (B2 and C1), retinol, copper peptides, and a vitamin and mineral complex. The active ingredients are delivered in a technologically advanced vehicle, in tiny microspheres called nanosomes, which are two hundred times smaller then human cells and penetrate into the deepest layers of the skin and release the active ingredients gradually over a fifteen-hour period. This technology dramatically boosts the effectiveness of the active ingredients, since they are absorbed much deeper in the skin.

Some less common treatments available online or overseas include these:

Dercos: This product, developed by L'Oréal Laboratories in France, contains a drug called aminexil. Researchers found that hair loss, no matter what its cause, is always accompanied by perifollicular fibrosis, a condition that causes the collagen around the root of the hair to become rigid and push the hair to the surface of the scalp. This condition may also affect the appearance and rapid disappearance of new hair follicles, as they can't be formed deep in the scalp. Aminexil has been shown to stop perifollicular fibrosis. Dercos is currently available in France and Germany and online at www.smart-drugs.net.

Folligen: This product is made up of copper peptides, potent free radical scavengers that act as both profound anti-inflammatory agents and antioxidants when applied directly to the scalp. The active copper peptides in Folligen have been shown to stimulate skin repair while possessing anti-inflammatory properties. Studies conducted at more than thirty leading universities and medical research institutes led by dermatologists and scientists have thoroughly established the effectiveness of the copper peptide technologies for hair and skin tissue regeneration. It may also be that these peptides inhibit the localized immune response responsible for so much hair loss, and may offset damage and inflammation already incurred. Unless the immunological factors involved in hair loss are dealt with, the potential for hair regrowth is limited.

Oz Garcia's MFR Solution: We have developed a lotion that has minoxidil, finasteride, and Retin-A in a solution that can be applied directly to the scalp. This has proved to be very effective for men (unlike Dercos and Folligen, this product can only used only by men). It can be ordered through our office in New York City.

Women don't usually experience total baldness, but they are prone to genetic alopecia, also known as female pattern hair loss (FPHL). For many women, hair loss or thinning seems to be triggered by menopause. This is extremely common; in fact, the Mayo Clinic estimates that about two-thirds of women face hair loss at some point during their lives. Again, no one knows the exact cause, but one theory says that when progesterone levels fall, the body responds by producing higher levels of androstenedione, a hormone with some "male-like" properties, including male pattern hair loss. Taking natural hormones like those discussed in chapter 10 can help restore hair growth. Hair growth is, however, a slow process, so you may not see results for four to six months.

Notes from Bruce Dean on Makeup

The way you apply makeup should change as you age. You evolve as a person, and so does your skin. I think it's important to go to a professional makeup artist and have your makeup done at least once a year, to revise your look and maybe change or modify a few things. Half the battle is having the right colors picked out for you. I see a lot of women wearing the wrong colors. Women who wear makeup well—who have a glow and look alive—wear the right colors for their skin.

Women often think that they should wear the same color eye shadow as their eyes. But if you have blue eyes and wear blue eye shadow, that blue eye shadow will actually compete with your eye color. If you want to bring out the blue in your eyes, wear warmer tones (the browns and rusts—but stay away from ash brown; it will mimic the dark circles under your eyes and make you look tired). Conversely, if you have warm brown eyes, you want to wear the cooler shades of blue to contrast with your eye color. That's the way to make your eyes pop.

The issue for women as they get older is skin quality. I've done makeup for women in their fifties who have incredible skin (they have a great diet, they're exercising, or they have really good genes—some women are just blessed). But most women need a little help. It's important to use the right techniques and makeup application for your face. I always say that a woman's makeup should be just as individual as her own fingerprint. My advice is to go to a makeup counter or a professional makeup artist and ask for help in choosing an appropriate foundation for your particular skin type. It's important to go every year because your skin changes as you get older. Many women find that their skin gets drier, but sometimes they experience the opposite. Go in, try new products, and find what works for your skin.

A good makeup artist will give you a more symmetrical face. It all comes down to symmetry, because that's what's attractive to people. For instance, if your eyes are too close together or too far apart, makeup can help you achieve a more balanced, symmetrical look.

One common mistake is to wear too much eyeliner and not enough mascara. I'd rather see less liner and more mascara to create a fuller lash. Another error women often make is wearing too much concealer. To avoid this, here's a tip: Apply eye makeup first, then the foundation, and the concealer last. Most women apply their foundation and concealer first, so that when they apply their eye makeup, they get those little crumbs that fall underneath the eye, which they try to cover up with more concealer. The result is that caked, lined, dry look. So do your eye makeup first and your foundation last. If you're using a powder foundation, use your concealer first because you shouldn't put a moist product over a dry one. But if you use liquid, do the foundation first and then the concealer. You might find that with the foundation under your eye, you'll need less concealer.

I enjoy working with clients who are willing to try something new—women who know themselves and their boundaries. That's important. Whenever someone is doing your makeup or your hair, it's important to speak up and let that person know what you like and what you don't like. The professional artist is there to help you. You should be working together to create this new version of yourself.

I became a makeup artist because I love to help people see themselves in a different way and feel more confident. When I do someone's face, it changes her perspective. She feels different. She approaches the world in a different way.

Notes from Dr. Marc Lowenberg on Veneers

In cosmetic dentistry, we can use several different techniques to brighten the teeth. There's bleaching or whitening. There's bonding, which is plastic resin that is sculpted on top of the teeth to change their shape or color. And then there are porcelain veneers, the technique in which I specialize.

A porcelain veneer is a laboratory-fabricated shell, very much like a fake fingernail, which is custom fitted to the patient's tooth. Placing veneers on the teeth changes their color, their shape, and their positioning. Veneers can give you that wide Julia Roberts megawatt smile, or elongate your front teeth to make them look more like Cindy Crawford's or Claudia Schiffer's. They can feminize or masculinize your teeth, as men tend to have more square-shaped teeth and women tend to have more rounded teeth.

Most people don't realize that as we get older, our teeth age just like every other part of the body. First of all, your teeth get darker as you get older—not necessarily yellower, but darker. If you have yellow teeth to begin with, they get more yellow. If you have gray-brown teeth, they will get more gray-brown. People often think their teeth are getting darker because they smoke cigarettes or drink a lot of coffee or tea, but those substances only stain your teeth on the surface; they don't change the intrinsic color of your teeth. Age is what changes the color of your teeth. One reason is that the enamel, the outer layer of the tooth structure, is translucent. As you get older you wear down the enamel just from brushing your teeth and eating food, or even from grinding your teeth. The thinner the enamel, the more translucent it is, and the more you see the color underneath the enamel. This layer of the tooth structure is called dentin, and it is almost always yellow or yellow-brown. If you have thicker enamel, you won't see as much of the yellow layer showing through.

Second, many years of eating, brushing, and grinding your teeth not only wears down the enamel but also tends to wear down or chip the edges of your teeth. This simply makes sense: If you've been biting into food for fifty years, your teeth are going to wear down.

Third, as we get older, the muscles around the mouth lose their tone and elasticity. Your upper lip tends to hang lower than it did when you were twenty years old. The lower lip, by force of gravity, also hangs lower. When that happens, you see less of your upper teeth and more of your lower teeth.

To rejuvenate your smile, you want to combat those three factors—color, worn-down edges, and the visibility of the lower teeth versus the upper teeth.

125

The best method for this is to use porcelain veneers, which will enable you to lengthen the top teeth and shorten the lower teeth as well as change their color. Then your smile can be tweaked in several ways.

The veneers are made by a ceramist, someone who specializes in porcelain. The ceramist takes into account all the patient's facial qualities: the shape of the face, the color of the skin, the wideness of the smile, and the color of the eyes and how they're set in the face. All these qualities come into play when you're designing somebody's smile.

When I first started my practice years ago, all my patients were women. Today, men make up 40 percent of my practice. Although most of those men tell me, "I'm here because my wife wants me to do my teeth," I recognize a generational trend. As we baby boomers have gotten older we have focused on changing the appearance of so many other parts of our bodies in order to look younger that many of us have neglected our teeth. In some ways, this is more of a problem for men than for women. Middle-aged men today, for instance, work out more than those of previous generations, but they tend not to think about how their teeth may be affecting their appearance. In fact, men's teeth tend to age and darken much more rapidly than those of their female counterparts, and since most men are not as delicate in their behavior as women, they're generally more prone to chipping or breaking their teeth. Also, they're generally not nearly as meticulous with their oral hygiene as women are, so their teeth tend to decay more, their gums become more inflamed, and the overall appearance of their teeth deteriorates much more rapidly.

But nowadays, you're held accountable for not having good teeth. Forty years ago, no one ever assumed that you would have good teeth when you got older. Today, in light of what we know about dental hygiene and the technology that's available in tooth care, there is every reason that you should have a bright, beautiful smile regardless of your age.

Veneers last for about fifteen to twenty years. That's because as you continue to age, your gums naturally recede. Since the veneers are made to your gum line, as your gums recede there will be a discrepancy between your gum and the veneer, at which point the veneer will tend to stain and chip and should be replaced. The good news is that getting veneers makes you look ten to fifteen years younger, because when you have a bright smile, people tend to notice that more so than any other feature of your face.

If you're looking for a dentist in your area to give you veneers, you should ideally choose someone on the basis of a referral from someone whose teeth have been veneered and look good to you. The best referral is from someone who can tell you what the procedure is like and what you can expect from the finished product. You should ask the dentist to describe to you what he or she would do to change your teeth. Have a clear understanding of what the dentist would do, and decide whether you would be happy with that.

Oz Wraps It Up

Remember this when you're having all these things done—getting veneers, coloring and styling your hair, and having your makeup done—whatever makes you feel good about yourself is generally worth doing, as long as you don't go to extremes (we've all heard stories of people who are addicted to plastic surgery). Pursuing beauty from the outside in, when done wisely, can do wonders for your confidence and self-esteem. Not only is looking good a result of staying healthy; it can be a great motivating factor to keep you on the right nutritional and exercise track as well.

127

PART IV

ALCHEMY:

EXPLORING THE BIOLOGICAL LANDSCAPE
OF AGE REVERSAL

THE "SCIENCE" OF alchemy was born in the Middle Ages. Its aims were to transmute base metals into gold, discover a universal cure for disease, and determine a means of prolonging life indefinitely. After all these years and despite all our knowledge, we are still in pursuit of alchemy. We persist in the search for a universal cure. We have already prolonged our lives considerably, and the research into human longevity continues apace.

Every day we break new boundaries in science and health that are changing how we use and apply medicine. Many of these breakthroughs occur in genomics (the study of organisms in terms of their DNA) and proteomics (the study of the structure, function, and interactions of proteins produced by the genes of a particular cell, tissue, or organism). Amazing things are on the horizon. We now have, for instance, the most comprehensive diagnostics imaginable that can tell you precisely how your body is functioning (this is discussed in chapter 9). Soon there will be proven medications and even vaccines to prevent obesity. We now know that you can use different versions of the RNA building blocks of the human body to slow down the development of diseases such as macular degeneration (the country's leading cause of blindness) as you get older. Scientists are pinpointing the genes that cause many diseases, and it won't be long before this knowledge is translated into cures and preventions. The way we will treat illnesses years from now is going to be very different from they way we treat them today.

However, we are not there yet. Pinpointing genes hasn't led to immediate help for those who are afflicted by disease. And as much as technology has advanced, it's not the answer to everything. In fact, according to an article titled "The Future of Medicine" by Geoffrey Cowley in the special "Health for Life" summer 2005 edition of *Newsweek*, "technological progress is not a complete recipe for better health, and there is real danger in equating newer with better. America has built the world's highest-tech medical system, yet the nation ranks forty-sixth in life expectancy (behind Japan, Singapore, Canada, and virtually all of Europe and Scandinavia). And forty-one countries, including Cuba, have achieved lower rates of infant mortality." In 2007, the United States had risen to number forty-two in life expectancy, still well behind other countries.

In other words, we can't rely on science to keep us healthy without taking some responsibility for ourselves. It's up to each one of us to investigate, compare notes, and seek out the best that science can offer to help us maintain the highest level of age efficiency possible.

If you want to live a long and healthy life, feel better, and be able to regulate the aging of your body—if you want to be transformed—you have to be informed. You have to know what's going on with your own body and what medicine can do for you at this point. That means not only having a dialogue with your mainstream doctor but also being aware of alternative practices and viewpoints, such as functional and environmental medicine (medical specialties that treat people from a wellness-based model as opposed to a disease-based model, and also treat problems that do not respond to conventional medical treatments). In the best of all possible worlds, you

will find a doctor who actually understands and incorporates several different models into his or her practice.

Over the years, I've developed professional relationships with several doctors and health professionals whose opinions I hold in high esteem and who are
among the leaders in antiaging medicine. We hear from some of them in this
part of the book, speaking on diverse subjects, from diagnostic testing to
menopause to pain care to brain maintenance. For these cutting-edge thinkers,
alchemy means "becoming"—using everything they know to help their patients become better versions of themselves.

NINE

DIAGNOSTICS

SEEING THE INSIDE STORY

THE WORD "DIAGNOSIS" comes from the Greek words *dia,* which means "by," and *gnosis*, which means "knowledge." Only through knowledge can we determine what's wrong and figure out how to make it right. For hundreds of years, people have gone to see health professionals when they've experienced some sign or symptom, whether it's as obvious as a bright red rash or as subtle as a loss of energy. In these cases, these professionals do their best to pinpoint the problem, suggest ways to eliminate it, and perhaps give advice on how to prevent it from happening again.

There is another side to diagnostics, however. Modern developments in science and technology have brought diagnostics to new levels of accuracy in identifying risk factors for disease and in detecting diseases that have no symptoms (at least in their beginning stages). Millions of lives have been saved because women—especially women in their fifties—have gotten mammograms, even though they had no outward sign of disease or discomfort. Hundreds of thousands of people are controlling the diabetes they didn't know they had until a simple diagnostic test made them aware of their disease. And we now have diagnostic tests for all kinds of genetic markers that tell us if we're in a particular group of people who are more likely than others to get various diseases. Some diagnostics are as simple as blood tests or urine samples, while others are highly complex technological advances, such as the Biophysical250 (see sidebar on page 146).

In this chapter, Dr. Richard Firshein, director of the Firshein Center for Comprehensive Medicine in New York City, a specialist in integrative approaches to wellness and longevity, and author of *Reversing Asthma* and *The Nutraceutical Revolution*, runs us through what he considers the diagnostic testing most necessary for the *Redesigning 50* program. Dr. Gottfried Kellerman, CEO of Neuroscience Inc., a company that produces nutritional supplements designed to boost and optimize neurotransmitter levels in the body, and Dr. Stephen Koch, clinical instructor at Mt. Sinai School of Medicine, talk about new developments in screening for neurotransmitter deficiencies and for heart disease.

Notes from Dr. Richard Firshein on Diagnostic Testing

For most people, especially women, fifty is an age of transition. It can and should be a very positive time of life, but it is also the time when a lot of changes happen. The biological clock tends to accelerate as many hormonal changes begin to occur. The good news is that when you reach your fifties, you can begin to test for these changes and then respond to them, and this gives you a much greater ability to control your biological destiny.

Obviously, you can't undergo every test listed here—you wouldn't have any blood left—but this will give you a sense of where you might want to focus your efforts. With your doctor or health professional, you can look at your specific symptoms or areas of concern, along with your medical and family history, and then prioritize the tests that might be most beneficial for you. When a patient comes to my office, I look at that patient's personal history, family history, previous laboratory tests, current health issues, concerns, and symptoms. Then we try to pinpoint the primary area of concern—whether it's fatigue, premature aging, or more specific medical problems. For instance, I might ask myself, *Is this a person who is prone to cancer or to heart disease? Is this a person who has longevity on his or her side, or has aging occurred much more rapidly?* Then we focus on the kinds of tests that will give us the information we need to go ahead with treatment, cure, and preventive techniques.

I have broken down the list of diagnostics below into what I consider first-tier and second-tier tests. First-tier tests are the basics that you must have—no question about it—to determine overall health and give you a baseline with which you can compare your results over the years. Second-tier tests are good to have but are not absolutely necessary unless you have specific health concerns.

First-Tier Tests

- *Cholesterol:* A simple blood test can tell you if you have elevated low-density lipoprotein (LDL), or "bad cholesterol." Your total cholesterol level should be less than 200 mg/dL (milligrams per deciliter). I consider 150 to 170 mg/dL to be the "safe level." According to the American Heart Association, there are three categories of total blood cholesterol levels:

  Desirable—Less than 200 mg/dL
  Borderline High Risk—200 to 239 mg/dL
  High Risk—240 mg/dL and above

  Your LDL cholesterol level greatly affects your risk of heart attack and stroke. The lower your LDL cholesterol, the lower your risk. In fact, this a better gauge of risk than total blood cholesterol. Your LDL cholesterol will fall into one of these categories:

  Optimal—Less than 100 mg/dL
  Near Optimal—100 to 129 mg/dL
  Borderline High—130 to 159 mg/dL
  High—160 to 189 mg/dL
  Very High—190 mg/dL and above

On its Web site (www.americanheart.org), the American Heart Association offers this explanation:

> When too much LDL cholesterol circulates in the blood, it can slowly build up in the inner walls of the arteries that feed the heart and brain. Together with other substances it can form plaque, a thick, hard deposit that can clog those arteries. . . . HDL cholesterol is known as the "good" cholesterol because a high level of it seems to protect against heart attack. Medical experts think that HDL tends to carry cholesterol away from the arteries and back to the liver, where it's passed from the body. Some experts believe that HDL removes excess cholesterol from plaque in arteries, thus slowing the buildup.

High-density lipoprotein (HDL) cholesterol levels should range from 40 to 50 mg/dL for the average man and from 50 to 60 mg/dL for the average woman. An HDL cholesterol that's less than 40 mg/dL is considered low and puts you at high risk for heart disease. Smoking, being overweight, and being sedentary can all result in lower HDL cholesterol.

If your total numbers (LDL + HDL) are significantly above 170 mg/dL, we take a closer look at the breakdown of the cholesterol. Often, I have patients come in and tell me, "My cholesterol is terrible. I just had it tested, and it's 220 or 230." When we do a breakdown of the HDL and the LDL, we might find that a significant portion of their cholesterol is good cholesterol, so their risk factor is actually quite low. That's an important consideration, because there's an overtendency to prescribe cholesterol-reducing drugs that patients take for the rest of their lives.

■ *Fasting Blood Glucose:* This blood glucose test, which is taken after you have not eaten for at least eight hours, measures the amount of glucose (sugar) in the blood. This test can be used to screen healthy, asymptomatic individuals for diabetes and prediabetes because diabetes is a common disease that begins with few, if any, symptoms. Results between 100 and 125 mg/dL indicate impaired glucose tolerance, also known as prediabetes. If you're in this category, you should have follow-up evaluations and testing. Results above 126 indicate the presence of diabetes. This test should be part of your yearly routine physical exam once you reach the age of forty-five to fifty, especially if you are at high risk for the development of diabetes because of a family history of the disease, if you are overweight, or both.

■ *Thyroid Testing:* Studies have shown that one out of eight women will experience some kind of thyroid problem, particularly as they get older. The thyroid is one of the body's most important glands. When it doesn't work properly, it can cause nervousness or fatigue, weaken the muscles, cause weight gain or loss, and impair memory. In earlier days, the thyroid was tested only when problems were presented. However, about thirteen million Americans—more of them women—are affected by a thyroid disease or disorder, according to the National Graves' Foundation. In fact, the Colorado Thyroid Disease Prevalence Study suggests that up to one in six people may have an underactive thyroid (hypothyroidism). Even if you don't have any symptoms (and since symptoms such as fatigue and weight gain or loss are often attributed to other factors), it's good to get your thyroid tested at least once before the age of fifty, then every few years until the age of sixty, and yearly after that.

■ *Liver and Kidney Function Tests:* LFTs (liver function tests) are a group of blood tests that can help show how well a person's liver is working. LFTs include measurements of albumin, various liver enzymes, cholesterol, and total protein. The liver filters metabolic waste products, excess sodium, and water from the blood, helping to eliminate them from the body. Along with the liver, the kidneys are another part of the waste-processing system of the body—urine goes from the kidneys into the bladder. The kidneys also help regulate blood pressure and the production of red blood cells. A simple yearly blood test can tell you whether both of these important organs are functioning at optimal levels.

■ *Bone Mineral Density (BMD) Testing:* This test, which determines the density of your bones, is used to screen for osteoporosis. It uses sound waves or small amounts of radiation, and your results are compared with the average BMD of a healthy young adult. A BMD test can detect bone loss at an early stage. Normal X-rays are not strong enough to detect bone loss until at least 30 percent of bone mass has been lost. You should have a baseline test done when you reach fifty—sooner if you have a history of fractures, or if you think you've lost height. If your bone density is low at the time of the screening, you should have it checked every year; otherwise, you can wait up to five years before repeating the test. BMD testing usually takes about five minutes, you don't need to undress for it, and no special preparation is necessary. There are several types of BMD tests, including the DXA scan and the standard X-ray test. If you're concerned about radiation (as I am), ultrasound bone scans are also available.

- *Pap Smear:* All women over the age of eighteen should have an annual Pap smear. One of the newer developments in this area is the ThinPrep Pap smear, which is the same as a regular Pap smear, except that instead of smearing cervical cells onto a slide, the doctor rinses the cells into a vial and sends it to a lab that filters out blood and mucus, which can potentially obscure cancerous cells. Some studies have shown this test to be 65 percent more effective in detecting abnormalities than the traditional Pap smear.

- *Human Papillomavirus (HPV) Test:* Another new recommended test is for the human papillomavirus (HPV). HPV infections are very common and most often remain asymptomatic. If symptoms do occur, they are usually manageable. Equally reassuring is the fact that condom use is likely to reduce the risk of infection. However, HPV can be an indicator of a risk for cervical cancer (you must have the virus to get cervical cancer, but you don't necessarily get cancer just because you have the virus). It is most prevalent among young, sexually active women, but anyone who is sexually active should have this test done at the same time as a Pap smear.

- *Mammograms:* After the age of forty, women should have mammograms every one to two years. If you have particularly dense breasts, which are more difficult to read by mammogram alone (ask your doctor about this), you might want to ask for a mammogram plus ultrasound. The ultrasound is a noninvasive procedure that uses sound waves to view the breast. MRI (magnetic resonance imaging) has also been proved effective for finding breast cancers; however, it is most appropriate for women who are at higher risk. MRI can also be effective for women who have very dense breasts or who have breast implants.

- *Colorectal Cancer Screening:* Colorectal cancer is the second leading cause of cancer death in the United States. If detected early, it has a good cure rate. There are several screening methods for this disease:

  - *Fecal Occult Blood Test (FOBT):* This is a stool test that looks for microscopic amounts of fecal blood. It is only 30 percent effective in detecting early cancer and should be performed once a year in conjunction with the other screening methods.

  - *Flexible Sigmoidoscopy:* An endoscope—a flexible tube with a light and camera on the end—is inserted into the rectum and lower third of the colon. This test checks for polyps, benign growths that can turn cancerous, and should be performed every five years.

  - *Colonoscopy:* This test is similar to the sigmoidoscopy except that it examines the entire colon. This process is done while the patient is under sedation and should be performed every ten years (more often if you have high risk factors such as a family history of colorectal cancer or a personal history of colitis or Crohn's disease).

Second-Tier Tests

- *Markers for Heart Disease:* High cholesterol is not the only important indicator for heart disease. In fact, other markers may be even more important, including C-reactive protein, homocysteine, fibrinogen, and lipoprotein (a). These risk factors are cumulative; the more you have, the greater your chances for the development of heart disease. The good news is that most of these markers can be detected by simple blood tests and controlled by following the New 50 Fusion Food Plan guidelines in chapter 1 and adding appropriate supplements.

- *Homocysteine*: Elevated levels of homocysteine have been linked to increased risk of premature coronary artery disease, stroke, and blood clots. High homocysteine levels can be controlled by taking vitamin B_6, vitamin B_{12}, and folic acid.

- *C-Reactive Protein (CRP)*: A sensitive marker of inflammation, this protein is released into the bloodstream any time there is active inflammation in the body caused by conditions such as fever, infection, or injury. A 1998 study showed that women with high levels of C-reactive protein had a fivefold increase in the risk for the development of cardiovascular disease, and a sevenfold increase in the risk for having a heart attack or stroke. As of now, there is no clear treatment for elevated levels of CRP. Since CRP is a marker of inflammation, usually caused by some kind of infection, it is thought that antibiotics may be an effective treatment. Studies are also under way to determine whether statin drugs, used to treat high cholesterol, may be useful in lowering CRP levels.

- *Fibrinogen*: This is a blood-clotting factor, which can cause hypercoagulation (the tendency of blood to clot as it moves through the body) and excessive blood thickening, both of which significantly increase your risk for heart attack or stroke. Studies have shown that fibrinogen levels go up as estrogen goes down. Therefore, estrogen replacement therapy (see chapter 10) can significantly reduce fibrinogen levels. High doses of fish oil, olive oil, vitamin A, and vitamin C have also been shown to reduce fibrinogen levels.

141

> • *Lipoprotein-Associated Phospholipase, or Lp(a)*: This is another marker, largely an inherited factor, which indicates the likelihood of inflammation of the heart and arteries. Lp(a) flows through the blood with LDL and is one of the components that makes LDL "bad." Unfortunately, however, lowering your LDL level does not always lower your level of Lp(a). As with fibrinogen, Lp(a) levels tend to increase as estrogen decreases. Some supplements that have been shown to lower Lp(a) levels include coenzyme Q10, vitamin C, and niacin.

■ *Metabolic Profile:* This group of tests delivers important information about the current status of your kidneys, liver, and electrolyte and acid/base balance as well as your blood sugar and blood proteins (some of the first-tier test may be part of this profile, such as glucose and liver and kidney function). It is routinely ordered as part of a blood workup for a medical exam or yearly physical. These tests will not necessarily pinpoint what is wrong, which is why abnormal test results are usually followed up with other specific tests to confirm or rule out a suspected diagnosis.

■ *Hormone Testing:* Usually, women in their late forties to fifties who have gone six months without a menstrual cycle are in menopause. Women's hormones play an increasing role in their health as they age. Low estrogen levels are associated with stress, headaches, and osteoporosis, while high estrogen levels increase the risk of breast cancer, especially in postmenopausal women. Hormonal tests can determine whether a woman is in perimenopause or menopause and also measure levels of estrogen, progesterone, and testosterone. While some women go through menopause with very few symptoms, for most women it's a time of very dramatic change, with symptoms such as dry skin, hair loss, loss of libido, vaginal dryness, weight gain, and changes in mental capacity. However, these symptoms are manageable once the hormone levels have been assessed.

BIOPHYSICAL250: THE ULTIMATE IN DIAGNOSTICS

The theory behind Biophysical250 is that anything that is wrong with you will show up in your blood. Your blood contains biomarkers, including proteins, enzymes, hormones, and other substances that can be measured and, if found to be elevated or depressed, may indicate the presence of various diseases.

This assessment measures 250 different biochemical markers that may indicate the presence of many conditions and diseases including cancer, cardiovascular disease, metabolic disorders, autoimmune disease, viral and bacterial diseases, and hormonal imbalance. In addition, the assessment provides a valuable baseline that enables individuals and physicians to monitor changes and trends in blood chemistry over time.

Biophysical250 is state-of-the-art health surveillance—at a state-of-the-art price. For all services, it costs $3400 (most health insurance companies do not yet cover the cost of this test). Biophysical will send someone to your home or office to draw your blood. In a few weeks, you will receive your own private, comprehensive report analyzing 250 biomarkers, along with a copy of the report for your physician. The report highlights any potential factors that require further scrutiny and gives a brief explanation of what they may indicate. You'll also receive a private phone consultation with a Biophysical physician who will review the results with you (and who, if you wish, will discuss the results with your personal physician).

143

- *Nutritional Testing:* This is a test for nutritional imbalance or deficiencies. It is often done in connection with symptoms such as fatigue and extreme vulnerability to colds, flus, and other illnesses as well as neurological problems such as numbness and tingling. Nutritional testing can be invaluable even for healthy people because almost all of us are born with inherited genetic weaknesses that cause us to be more prone to certain illnesses. It will determine factors such as mineral, zinc, vitamin C, and calcium deficiencies; a stressed nervous system; malabsorption problems; adrenals that are fatigued or exhausted; and too many harmful bacteria in the intestines.

- *Digestive Testing:* Poor digestion can lead to gas and bloating, abdominal pain, diarrhea, constipation, food allergies, production of toxins, increased risk of colon cancer, and increased risk of ulcerative colitis. This test takes a comprehensive look at the gastrointestinal tract, offering information about digestion, absorption, bacterial balance, yeast overgrowth, inflammation, metabolic activity, and immune function.

Notes from Dr. Stephen Koch on the Importance of Cardiac CT Angiography for Women

The newest development in the detection of heart disease is cardiac CT angiography (CTA). Diagnosing heart disease as early as possible is vital because heart disease is the number one killer of both men and women in the United States. It kills more people each year than all other causes of death combined, including all forms of cancer. While cardiac CT angiography is useful for everyone, it is particularly important for women for several reasons:

- Most women do not consider themselves to be at great risk for heart disease.
- While 25 percent of men who have heart attacks die within a year, more than 38 percent of women die within that same time frame.
- 63 percent of women who die from heart disease had no previous symptoms.
- Some diagnostic tests and procedures, including the exercise stress test or stress ECG, are less accurate in women than in men.
- Many women do not recognize the early signs of a heart attack. Women may experience early symptoms of cardiovascular disease

differently than men. The symptoms in women can be far subtler.
They may include

- Shortness of breath, often without chest pain of any kind
- Flulike symptoms—specifically nausea, clamminess, or
  cold sweats
- Unexplained fatigue, weakness, or dizziness
- Pain in the chest, upper back, shoulders, neck, or jaw
- Feelings of anxiety, loss of appetite, discomfort

If you even suspect these symptoms, call your doctor or 911, or go to a local
hospital's emergency room.

Heart disease is also the single most preventable cause of death. The lifestyle choices we make—such as smoking, failing to get regular exercise, and
eating unhealthy foods—can significantly increase the risk of heart disease.
Making healthier choices dramatically reduces those risks.

Heart disease becomes an even greater problem for women after menopause. Estrogen helps protect women from heart disease, so when the ovaries
stop producing estrogen, the risk of heart disease increases dramatically. While
breast cancer is the disease most women fear the most, the truth is that heart
disease and strokes produce the most fatalities. Every sixty seconds, someone
in this country suffers a fatal heart attack. Half of those persons have had no
warning and no previous symptoms.

That's why this new technology of cardiac CT angiography is so important. Standard stress tests don't show any abnormalities until an artery is at
least 60 percent narrowed. Most heart attacks occur in arteries that are less
than 50 percent narrowed and therefore not detectable by any form of stress
testing.

Cardiac CT angiography is a revolutionary method of visualizing the
inside of the coronary arteries. It can create amazingly detailed and accurate
images of the heart, lungs, and arteries in just seconds. It's a ten- to
fifteen-second exam that has the capability of changing people's lives by identifying a disease that might never show a sign or symptom for another fifteen

or twenty years. When detected early, chances are good that the progression of the disease can be halted or even reversed and heart attacks or strokes can be prevented.

Women forty-five to sixty years old, as a demographic, generally aren't individuals with long-standing disease, but they are developing low-density soft plaques (the earliest form of calcium buildup in the arteries of the heart), which are difficult to detect with traditional testing. CTA technology, however, has been proved to have a very high positive and negative predictive value—meaning that if disease is there, you're going to see it, and if it's not there, you'll be able to see that as well.

With this donut-shaped machine (as opposed to the tube shape of an MRI device), the CTA can image the chest or any anatomic location in an extremely short time. Because it takes just a few seconds, it can capture the heart in stop-motion, which is the key to being able to see and pinpoint damaged areas.

Another important point about women and heart disease is that, as mentioned, their symptoms are not the typical crushing chest pains, which makes heart disease in women more difficult to diagnose. That's why the CTA is especially good for women.

Notes from Dr. Gottfried Kellerman on Neurotransmitter Testing

Most people have heard the term "neurotransmitters" but don't know how they relate to our health; how they affect our moods, temperament, and ability to think; or how they influence the aging process. Until very recently, most doctors—whether traditional or alternative—have taken the nervous system for granted, assuming that it runs perfectly well all the time. But the fact is that the nervous system, like everything else in the body, declines with time and age. Consequently, something needs to be done about it.

DEFINING NEUROTRANSMITTERS

Neurotransmitters are chemicals that allow the movement of information from one neuron (a type of cell found in the brain and body that is designed to process and transmit information) across the gap, or synapse, between it and an adjacent neuron. After they cross the synapse, neurotransmitters are accepted by the next neuron at a specialized site called a receptor.

The first neurotransmitter was discovered in 1921. Since then, many neurotransmitters have been discovered, including acetylcholine (particularly important in the stimulation of muscle tissue), epinephrine (adrenaline) and norepinephrine (compounds secreted principally from the adrenal gland that can cause increased heart rate and the enhanced production of glucose for the fight-or-flight response), dopamine (which facilitates critical brain functions and, when overproduced, may play a role in Parkinson's disease, certain addictions, and schizophrenia), serotonin (assumed to play a biochemical role in mood and mood disorders, including anxiety, depression, and bipolar disorder), and insulin (a peptide secreted by the pancreas that stimulates other cells to absorb glucose).

147

These days, our hectic lifestyles take a terrible toll on the nervous system. We're typically in highly demanding, high-stress situations. And stress situations are clearly linked to the nervous system. What we see in the "middle-aging" population are serious deficiencies in several neurotransmitters, primarily in serotonin. These deficiencies can cause a variety of symptoms to which we can all relate, including insomnia and increased nervousness, agitation, and anxiety.

We have developed a means of testing the levels of transmitters in both urine and saliva, so that we're able to get a complete landscape of what's going on in the body.

The nervous system consists of two parts: central and peripheral. When people think of neurotransmitters, they think mostly of mental functions, but that's a misconception. The nervous system is just as important in its peripheral functions. Our heart rate is controlled by neurotransmitters, as is our digestion, so all kinds of seemingly unrelated problems may actually be linked to neurotransmitters. That's why almost everybody who is approaching middle age can benefit from this kind of testing. We have found that up to 90 percent of all middle-aged people have deficient or suboptimal neurotransmitter levels.

Currently, we're able to test for ten to fifteen of the most important neurotransmitters. Here are just a few of them:

- *Serotonin:* The overall governing neurotransmitter that affects emotions, behavior, and thought.
- *Dopamine:* It has been linked to the pleasure center of the brain, but it has also been proved to link to several important gastrointestinal functions.
- *Phenylethylamine (PEA):* It has been called the love neurotransmitter because people who are in love have high PEA levels. PEA is also very much involved in cognitive function.
- *Glutamate:* It is involved in cognitive function, in terms of the way you think and feel.

One of the most important contributions we have made in this field is to establish optimal levels for neurotransmitters. Although some neurotransmitter testing has been around for twenty to thirty years, guidelines were missing under which nervous system functions could be measured for optimal levels. We have established these guidelines. This was accomplished by selecting three hundred healthy men and women, ages twenty-five to thirty-five. The selection criteria were that they were in their prime, had no clinical or medical complaints, were free of medication, and generally felt great. We took neurotransmitter levels from those "ideal" people and determined that if they function so well—if they're healthy and happy—then those levels would give us a baseline to compare with those of people who are getting older or have problems. Accordingly, we adjust or correct the neurotransmitter levels of patients to match that baseline.

One interesting discovery is that there is no gender difference in neurotransmitter levels. We did not find any significant differences between men and women in terms of the decline of their nervous systems. Our database, which has processed the test results of more than one hundred thousand people so far, has shown us that the old wives' tale that women have lower levels of serotonin is just not true.

Once you get your report back, you will be able to see the results and get a sense of where you have age-related problems and what you can do to begin to correct those neurotransmitter levels. Generally, this "normalization" is done through medication, but many people choose to take a progressive approach instead. For example, they may opt to begin by following something like the *Redesigning 50* program, adjusting their diet and their lifestyle, and incorporating the therapeutic use of nutraceuticals (supplements)—particularly amino acids.

Many neurotransmitters are made in the body from very simple amino acid precursors. The major precursors are common amino acids such as tyrosine, which makes adrenaline, noradrenaline, and dopamine. Serotonin is made from L-tryptophan. These are all amino acids that are contained in our daily diet, as long as we eat in accordance with a program like the New 50 Fusion Food Plan. The body is constantly breaking down and digesting proteins, which are made from amino acids; so if you get enough protein in your diet, you should theoretically be making enough neurotransmitters.

However, many people—especially younger people—tend to live mainly on carbohydrates, and carbohydrates do not contain the precursors needed to make neurotransmitters. This is how most of us get into trouble when we're younger, and by the time we reach middle age, the casualties are much higher. That's why I recommend that you add nutraceuticals to support the nervous system (see chapter 13).

Let me add one more important point. The nervous system is extremely complex and consists of many interactive neurotransmitters. Consequently, if you start correcting one neurotransmitter, it might have an effect on a second or third or fourth neurotransmitter as well. That's why if you feel a little bit

149

depressed or you have problems with your digestion, it doesn't make sense to test for only one neurotransmitter. You need to test for at least six or eight neurotransmitters to get a good idea of what might be wrong.

Unfortunately, many doctors still lack education in this area. When patients come in complaining about insomnia, moodiness, PMS (premenstrual syndrome), or depression, not many doctors will think in terms of neurotransmitter abnormalities or recognize that the imbalance could be within the brain. As a result, doctors have been quick to prescribe antidepressants, which are medications related to the correction of neurotransmitters, without prescribing adequate testing. My hope is that we will come to the point where neurotransmitter testing becomes part of a routine workup, in which we check your thyroid, we check your cholesterol, and we check your neurotransmitters. This is what we are trying to accomplish. In the meantime, the push for neurotransmitter testing may have to come from patients, not necessarily from doctors.

We're not advocating that people stop their medication; in fact, these medications work well for many people. We do suggest testing to see whether other more progressive choices, such as the use of amino acid supplements, could work as well to bring neurotransmitter levels back to where they were when you were in your thirties.

Oz Wraps It Up

Some diagnostic tests are routinely given by most doctors; others are not part of traditional medicine's paradigm, and it may be up to you to inquire about many of these tests. If you're interested in healthy aging, it's important to take a baseline approach—to know where you are, healthwise, at any given point in time. You need to measure your health as precisely as possible and then do whatever is necessary to either maintain your status quo or correct and repair whatever problems you may find.

THE ESTROGEN/ TESTOSTERONE QUESTION

DISCUSSING HORMONE HEALTH, MENOPAUSE, AND ANDROPAUSE

MOST WOMEN DREAD menopause. They may have symptoms for as long as ten years before menopause even starts; this phase of a woman's life is known as perimenopause. Both perimenopause and menopause are stages in a lengthy process called the climacteric, which may begin for women as early as the age of thirty-five and as late as age sixty.

At any point during this process, women may experience hot flashes, vaginal dryness, mood swings, night sweats, and often lowered sex drive. Some fortunate women will have no symptoms whatsoever and will wonder what all the fuss is about. Others will experience all these discomforts and wonder how they can get through it. Most women will fall somewhere in the middle.

In this chapter, we hear from three experts in the fields of hormones, women's health, and issues surrounding menopause: Dr. Jeffrey I. Mechanick, endocrinologist and director of the Metabolic Support Service at Mt. Sinai School of Medicine in New York City; Dr. Erika Schwartz, renowned women's health advocate, expert in bioidentical hormones, and bestselling author of *The Hormone Solution* and *The 30-Day Natural Hormone Plan*; and Dr. Jeffrey Morrison, director of the Morrison Center in New York City and practitioner of integrative and environmental medicine. We also learn about andropause, the decline in testosterone that affects men in middle age, and the ever-prevalent subject of erectile dysfunction.

Notes from Dr. Jeffrey Mechanick
on Understanding Menopause

The word I hear most from women who come to me with symptoms of menopause is "confusion." They want to relieve their symptoms but have heard several different opinions on how best to treat them. The average woman with menopausal symptoms is bewildered by the lack of general consensus among physicians about how to deal with this ubiquitous problem. A gynecologist might discourage the use of any hormone replacement therapy, while another doctor might say it's okay to take estrogen but in a much smaller dose than used to be prescribed five to ten years ago. Someone else might say it's okay to take a larger dose of estrogen for a short time until the hot flashes get better. What is a woman supposed to do with this conflicting information?

Physicians are also frustrated because the issue has never really been settled, even after the 2002 Women's Health Initiative (WHI) study. At that time, more than six million American women were taking a combination of estrogen and progesterone to treat symptoms of menopause. After the WHI study found that the combined drugs caused increases in breast cancer, heart attacks, strokes, and blood clots, many doctors switched to prescribing estrogen alone. Some doctors take the hard-line view that you still shouldn't take estrogen because you're at increased risk for the conditions mentioned above; others take the opposite view and believe that it's okay to take estrogen; still others take an intermediate view—which is where I find myself—that the relative risks increase when you have a first-degree relative who had breast cancer or if you yourself have already had breast cancer. In this last case, the menopausal symptoms would have to be really severe to make the risks of taking estrogen worthwhile.

As I look at it, if a woman in early menopause is having debilitating symptoms, and she herself doesn't have or hasn't had breast cancer, then it is probably all right for her to take low-dose estrogen—the lowest dose of estrogen necessary to treat those symptoms—with the understanding that it will be a lower-than-standard dose and will only be temporary, meaning six months to a year.

It often helps patients deal with the symptoms of menopause when they understand what's going on in their bodies. One of the most common symptoms is the hot flash. For many women, the symptoms of menopause begin with the hot flash, which is a vasomotor reflex. You have neurons in a part of the brain called the hypothalamus, which controls the pituitary gland, known as the master gland. The hypothalamus contains a variety of neurons that control mechanisms, which in turn control blood vessels and blood flow. These neurons are influenced by estrogen. When you reduce or remove the estrogen, the neurons become hyperactive and begin to produce chemicals that are similar to adrenaline. This hyperactivity causes vasomotor instability: the blood vessels dilate, there's more blood flow, and you get the temporary sensations of heat, flushing, and sweating.

Another typical symptom of menopause is night sweats. No one is precisely sure why women experience night sweats, but it may be related to the fact that our bodies abide by a circadian rhythm (*circa* means "around," and *dian* means "day"). Over the course of a twenty-four-hour day, certain hormones peak at certain times of the day. Thyroid hormones and cortisol (an adrenal hormone), for instance, tend to rise in the early morning. Night sweats are probably related to the normal changes in hormones that occur during sleep, predisposing or creating an environment where the hot flash can occur.

A fair amount of data link estrogen with several cognitive dysfunction and neurodegenerative diseases such as Alzheimer's. The brain is what we term sexually dimorphic, meaning that during embryology and development of the brain, it develops one way under the influence of estrogen and another way if not as much estrogen is present. If you look at some of the standardized testing of young children, girls and boys often test differently, and this difference is thought to be due to the influence of sex steroids. Therefore, it is plausible that during menopause, when you have the withdrawal of estrogen, there may be neurological, psychiatric, and cognitive changes that will show up more in some women than in others because of genetic differences and sensitivities.

153

LOSS OF LIBIDO

A common complaint among women who are going through menopause is a loss of libido. This may be due to the natural decrease in testosterone that occurs as women age. According to www.womenshealth.com, along with the decrease of estrogen and progesterone that occurs during menopause, women "also slightly decrease production of testosterone. The word *slightly* is important here because the lower amount of testosterone is less important than the fact that the ratio of testosterone to estrogen and progesterone changes."

Many studies have shown a positive connection between testosterone supplementation and an increased level of sexual desire, energy, and general well-being in women. Of course, as with everything else, testosterone supplementation has possible side effects, including weight gain, acne, oily skin, excess body hair, or other masculinizing effects. A recent study showed that women taking a low-dose estrogen-testosterone combination reported a twofold improvement in sexual interest, compared with women who were taking estrogen alone.

A report published in the journal *Menopause* by the North American Menopause Society (NAMS) in 2005 ("The Role of Testosterone Therapy in Postmenopausal Women") stated that testosterone "has a positive effect on sexual function, primarily desire, arousal, and orgasmic response, in women after spontaneous or surgically induced menopause." The same report stated that the U.S. Food and Drug Administration (FDA) recommends testosterone for postmenopausal women with diminished sexual function, but it says this advice applies only to women taking concurrent estrogen therapy. Not enough evidence exists to make recommendations for women who are not taking estrogen or for those who wish to use testosterone therapy for longer than six months.

There is no one-size-fits-all solution for loss of libido. Women who are willing to try testosterone therapy may have to go through a trial-and-error period with their health-care professional to find the dose that is best for them.

Notes from Dr. Erika Schwartz
on Bioidentical Hormones

The first thing you need for surviving menopause is a doctor who listens to you, who cares about you, and who is willing to put all the pieces together and be your coach and your advocate. If your doctor understands diet, exercise, and nutrition and wants to help you, you're in good shape.

It's not always easy to find a doctor like that. And it's not always easy to find a doctor who is knowledgeable about hormones and hormone imbalances. To some extent, it's your responsibility to educate yourself and to understand that hormones affect everything you do. Hormones are powerful agents of change in your body. They cause direct changes in bodily functions and also facilitate your body's reaction to changes in the world around you. And this goes for everyone—men, women, children, adolescents, senior citizens.

When our hormones are out of balance, problems can develop. Our skin gets dry and wrinkled, we develop insomnia, we gain weight, and we lose interest in sex. Our joints ache. We get osteoporosis, digestive problems, and heart disease. We age prematurely.

Since we know that the production of certain hormones decreases when we hit menopause, we can easily conclude that this is a time when hormones are out of balance. That's why hormone replacement therapy came into practice. However, the synthetic hormones that were used as replacements turned out to involve high-risk factors. The good news is that there are now alternatives. They are called natural, or bioidentical, hormones, meaning that they are biologically identical to human hormones. They are precise duplications of the estrogen and progesterone produced by the human female reproductive system. The molecular structure of these hormones, which are made from plants such as yams and soy, is indistinguishable from that of the natural hormones produced in the body. Because the body "sees" them as exactly like the hormones that are already there, they are less likely to cause adverse reactions.

ON NATURAL HORMONES

I started seeing Erika Schwartz when I was in my midforties. I'm fifty-one, and I'm still getting my period every month. When I first saw Erika, though, I was going through some changes. My period was getting heavier. I was getting moodier. I've always preferred to go with early prevention rather than waiting until something happens and then going to see a doctor. So I went to see Erika. She put me on the natural hormones, and I've been taking them ever since.

I went because I felt that my periods were changing. I guess I was in perimenopause, which you can be in for years. I never wanted to go the conventional route with hormone replacement therapy because I've read too many things about the risk of cancer. There are so many drugs you take thinking that you're doing the right thing, and then years later you find out it was the worst thing you could have taken for yourself and for your children. I've always been inclined to take the natural approach.

When I first spoke to Erika, I wasn't sure if I should start on the natural hormones or if this was something I should hold off on. Erika put me on small doses of progesterone and testosterone. And every couple of months I go to see her for a blood test to see if the hormone levels are changing. Of course, I also see a gynecologist yearly for the regular mammograms and Pap smears. I'm not going through any of the symptoms of hot flashes or cravings or weight gain.

Of course, a lot has to do with your genetic makeup. My mom never took any medication, and she never had hot flashes or anything like that—just one day she didn't have her periods anymore. But there's a lot you can do even if you haven't been dealt the best hand genetically. There's so much you can do to keep yourself healthy.

RICKI LUBART, FIFTY-ONE,
MARRIED, MOTHER

Also, unlike synthetic hormones, bioidentical hormones are tailored to a patient's unique physiology and needs, and the prescription is then formulated by a compounding pharmacy. When the effects are known, the formulation can be fine-tuned or adjusted until the patient attains optimal relief.

Notes from Dr. Jeffrey Morrison on Women's Health

I practice what is now called integrative medicine, which means that I am able to combine the best of conventional medicine with everything I've learned in what was once called alternative medicine but is now known as complementary medicine. Because we integrate the best of both worlds, I have many different options at my disposal to help bring people to a better state of health and well-being.

Many of my patients are women in their fifties who are beginning to experience perimenopause or menopause. One of their biggest complaints is that they just don't have the energy they used to have. After I assess their history and give them a physical exam, I determine what blood tests are needed to establish whether there are any nutritional deficiencies. After I get the results of these tests, I can prescribe nutritional treatment to correct the problems.

When we are young, our body is extremely efficient at healing itself. As we get older and experience the damaging effects of time and exposure to toxins of all kinds, our bodies cannot work as efficiently. Things start to break down and do not repair themselves. The good news is that we can completely reverse the damage if we get to it before it's too late. We begin by looking at the basics and giving the body the proper environment for it to heal itself. We do this by providing a high-quality diet, proper nutrients, exercise, bioidentical hormones, and detoxification.

When women come to see me, they are ready to make a big change in their lives. What I want to do initially is help them begin to reduce inflammation and get rid of water retention. I start them on a short-term detoxification fast. Some of the nutrients that I use to detox are Liv52 (two to three tablets twice a day), an amino acid called N-acetyl-cysteine (1,000 milligrams twice a day), a nutrient called alpha-lipoic acid, or ALA (100 milligrams twice a day), and glutathione (1,000 milligrams twice a day).

I then recommend a longer-term food plan that leans heavily on the Mediterranean-style diet. My patients get really motivated when they see that they can lose weight very quickly on this diet. Their energy increases because

157

their bodies are detoxifying and are no longer overloaded with so many poor-quality foods. With the proper diet, the body will start working properly.

It's also extremely important to take antioxidants to fight off all the damage that's been done over the years. One of the best antioxidants is vitamin C. Intravenous vitamin C treatment especially is a very powerful way to help improve the way the body handles many different aspects of health. It helps protect the immune system, improve insulin sensitivity, and recharge the adrenal gland, which helps the body deal with stress. It also helps improve energy so women are able to exercise more efficiently, effectively, and for longer durations of time. You really can't get this benefit from taking vitamin C pills. If you take vitamin C orally, you're able to absorb only about 6,000 milligrams. Intravenous vitamin C is given in very high doses (under medical supervision, of course), often between 25,000 and 100,000 milligrams. (You can find out about other important antioxidants in chapter 13.)

We take a global approach to keeping the whole body in balance so that it continues to work effectively and efficiently. That's why we include exercise in our program, as well as nutritional factors. One thing we've forgotten in the modern world is that we are not meant to sit in one place all day. Just moving our bodies makes us feel better. When we move, it stimulates and increases our heart rate; it allows our circulation to reach all the different parts of the body; our blood vessels open up and are more receptive to all the nutrients our body is consuming; and our different gland systems rev up to meet the demands that we're putting on our body.

The old saying really is true: If you don't use it, you lose it. It's like putting your car in the garage. If you leave it sitting there for ten years, there's no way you'll be able to start that thing up. But if you run it every single day, you can run it for one or two hundred thousand miles. If you use good-quality fuel, change the spark plugs, and rotate the tires, it will run for quite a long time. The human body is a similar machine in that we have to take care of it—for example, by fueling it with high-quality nutrients and "running the engine" on a regular basis. It's the best way I know to live a long, healthy, vital life.

Andropause: Hormone Changes and the Male Menopause

One of the biggest problems for men in their forties and fifties is the change in testosterone (the primary male hormone), in particular the levels of free testosterone circulating in the blood (approximately 2 percent of total testosterone is made up of free testosterone; the rest is attached to proteins in the blood). This decline is called andropause and is sometimes referred to as the male menopause. Andropause is not as dramatic an event as menopause. There isn't any "pause," as there is for women who stop menstruating. But there is a syndrome in which several different bodily functions slow down and noticeable changes in the male body begin to take place.

Here's a quick run-through of what happens as men age: declining levels of testosterone begin to contribute to abdominal weight gain; loss of lean body mass; a decline in energy, strength, and stamina; depression; elevated cholesterol; and other conditions associated with aging. Degenerative diseases such as heart disease, stroke, diabetes, arthritis, osteoporosis, and hypertension are also linked directly or indirectly to testosterone decline.

Part of this aging is a kind of "feminizing effect" as male estrogen levels begin to increase, blocking the ability of testosterone to work effectively in the brain, nerves, muscles, and genitals. It is important to keep testosterone in the free form in our bloodstream to activate the proper cell receptors that affect the libido.

If you are a man and are concerned about your diminished sex drive, you should first see your doctor and get tested. You need the proper blood work to determine whether low levels of both free and total testosterone are at the root of your problem. It's a well-documented fact that middle-aged men with a testosterone deficit often have difficulty getting aroused and/or staying aroused long enough to enjoy having sex. Sexual arousal begins in your brain, where the neuronal testosterone receptors are stimulated by the presence of the hormone. If inadequate amounts of testosterone are present, arousal will not occur.

Once you've determined that your hormone levels are low, there are several ways to normalize them, to bring them back to acceptable levels. It is possible to use synthetic testosterone prescribed by your doctor, but a better method

159

might be to use natural testosterone such as Androderm, which is available in patch form and is approved by the FDA for men with insufficient levels of testosterone.

A second line of support is to use nutraceuticals that contain dietary nutrients known to block undesirable levels of estrogen in men and to increase levels of desirable free testosterone:

- *Chrysin:* This is a plant extract known as bioflavonoid that blocks aromatase, the enzyme that triggers testosterone conversion into estrogen. The less testosterone that is converted, the more is available for to you. Chrysin is added to many products used by bodybuilders as part of their muscle fitness programs. It is also a potent antioxidant, has been shown to reduce inflammation, and may also play a role in moderating the undesirable effects of stress hormones in the body. This plant compound appears to work best in the presence of piperine (an extract of pepper) or other plant-based bioflavonoids. I recommend a nutraceutical formula by Life Extension Foundation (LEF) called MiraForte with Chrysin. LEF has conducted extensive studies on its formulation, which includes several additional herbs such as nettles and muira puama.

- *Nettles:* This herb works by inhibiting the form of testosterone known as DHT in the blood, which can lead to premature hair loss and prostate enlargement. It also controls the levels of sex hormone binding globulin (SHBG), which renders free testosterone inactive.

- *Muira puama:* This is a libido enhancer that comes from the stems and roots of a plant found in the Amazon region of South America. It has been the subject of two published clinical studies conducted by Dr. Jacques Waynberg of the Institute of Sexology in Paris, France, and was discussed as far back as 1994 in the *American Journal of Natural Medicine.* The studies outline the broad impact of muira puama on a range of parameters affecting sexual function, including the inability to maintain an erection. Various manufacturers currently market it as a natural Viagra. Muira seems to work by favorably altering the hormone balance in the aging male. It also seems to reverse much of the physical discomfort associated with lower levels of testosterone, including fatigue, loss of strength, and weakened sexual performance.

The Future of Sexual Performance: Viagra and Beyond

Scientists are currently studying several drugs and combinations of drugs that work in the brain and produce the best local effect—a cocktail of sorts that would affect the pleasure centers in the brain and increase localized sensation in the genital area. Let's look at a few available products:

- *Viagra:* It's hard to imagine anyone in the world who hasn't heard of Viagra. Many men who were previously embarrassed to bring up the subject of erectile dysfunction with their doctors are suddenly eager to ask for Viagra. In fact, in the few years since Pfizer introduced Viagra, it has become one of the biggest-selling drugs in history. Viagra increases a naturally produced enzyme called cyclic GMP (guanosine monophosphate), which is essential to maintaining an erection in men and increasing genital sensitivity in women. Rather than increasing desire or appetite for sex, it increases sensation on a local level. Viagra does have its side effects. Some patients have reported congestion, diarrhea, facial flushing, and headaches. A small percentage of men have also reported temporary changes in their vision, including sensitivity to light and a bluish tinge in their vision. According to an article by Reuters that appeared on July 9, 2005, in the *New York Times* ("Viagra Label to Note Risk of Vision Loss"), the U.S. Food and Drug Administration approved new labeling for Viagra, Cialis, and Levitra—the three most popular drugs for erectile dysfunction—to warn men about a possible link

161

of these drugs to a rare form of blindness. And men with heart disease, especially those who take nitroglycerin medication, are advised never to take Viagra.

- *Verdenafil (brand name Levitra):* This is Bayer's foray into the prosexual drug market. It works similarly to Viagra by inhibiting PDE-5, an enzyme that stops cyclic GMP from doing its job. It may have a slight edge on Viagra, since the studies indicate that more men using this drug were able to complete sexual intercourse all the way to ejaculation. It seems to be somewhat more selective than Viagra at targeting the PDE-5 enzyme and works better at lower doses.

- *Alpha MSH or PT 141:* This prosexual drug, originally called Melanotan, comes out of the University of Arizona. It was intended to produce a nice tan and help reduce skin cancer. While it does produce a beautiful tan, it also produces spontaneous erections. It has a very high success rate and appears to affect both desire and physical performance. Researchers believe that the drug acts specifically on a part of the brain known as the hypothalamus, setting off the arousal centers there.

- *Alprostadil:* Commercially known as Caverjet, this drug is a prostaglandin preparation that is prescribed by a doctor and used by direct injection into the penis. It works by relaxing the smooth muscle of the penis and the muscles surrounding the arteries, allowing an increase in blood flow through the cavernosal arteries, engorging them and creating an erection. A study published in the March 2001 issue of *Urology* showed that 85 percent of seventy men with erectile dysfunction who used Caverjet over a twelve-month period showed a return of spontaneous erections. Topiglan, a topical gel version of this product (and probably the one most men would prefer), is also available from your doctor.

- *Apromorphine or Uprima:* Uprima was initially investigated as a possible drug for Parkinson's disease. Unlike Viagra, which acts directly on blood flow to the penis, Uprima sparks an erection by stimulating a brain chemical related to arousal. This drug may work well for people with compromised health issues, such as high blood pressure or diabetes, who are facing significant levels of erectile dysfunction. It's also an option for men with heart disease who can't use Viagra. Several studies have been done on this medication showing that Uprima works in the part of the brain where the neurosignaling takes place. The drug assists the brain in converting the desire to have an erection into the actual mechanisms involved in producing one. It's extremely fast acting—ten minutes as opposed to Viagra's one hour. This drug, however, has not yet been approved by the FDA.

Oz Wraps It Up

Aging precipitates major changes in sexual function for both men and women. That doesn't mean you become asexual as you get older. There's no reason you shouldn't continue to enjoy a robust sex life for as long as you wish, especially with the ongoing scientific advances in the field of human sexuality. You may not be able to perform as well as you could when you were in your twenties or thirties. And it's true that as you get older, health and fitness issues play central roles in your sexual experience—poor nutrition, being out of shape, and too much stress can all take a toll on your sexual ability and enjoyment. So if you want to maintain a healthy, active sexuality throughout your life (and who doesn't?), you have to keep the big health picture in mind.

163

ELEVEN

ACHING AND AGING

ALTERNATIVES IN PAIN CARE

A FRIEND AND I were recently talking about getting older, and she told me that, for the most part, she didn't mind adding on the years. The one thing that did bother her, she said, was waking up every morning wondering what part of her body was going to ache that day. Aching seems to be the most common complaint about getting older. And it seems to start the day we turn fifty and head downhill from there. Knees, hips, feet, shoulders, wrists, fingers—name a body part, and at some point it begins to ache.

Aches and pains may come with age, but that doesn't mean you simply have to live with them. Many aches and pains come from inflammation in the joints and other parts of the body. One of the biggest problems we face as we age is inflammatory damage to the body. There is a highly inflammatory compound in our cells called nuclear factor kappa B (NFkB). Any number of things can increase the production and activity of NFkB, including poor nutrition, too much sun exposure, and especially free radical damage. You can reduce inflammation in several ways—beginning by following the New 50 Fusion Food Plan, which is rich in omega-3 fatty acids and naturally occurring antioxidants found in fruits and vegetables.

Of course, keeping yourself in the best physical shape possible by exercising regularly and using nutraceuticals such as alpha-lipoic acid, MSM (methylsulfo-nylmethane), and silica (which we learn about in chapter 13) can help ward off aches and pains as well.

However, even when we follow the best food, exercise, and nutraceutical plan, we can't avoid pain altogether. No matter how careful we are, the body experiences a certain amount of inevitable wear and tear from daily activities that may cause varying degrees of pain, not to mention pain brought on by illness or injury. The good news is that many helpful options are available to deal with pain. In this chapter we hear from three experts about four different methods of pain relief: Dr. John Juhl, osteopath and practicing member of the Ostrow Institute for Pain Management; Albert Garcia, massage therapist and cofounder of the Longevity Lounge and RestoreSpa (and, coincidentally, my brother and business partner); chiropractor Dr. Daniel Fenster; and physical therapist Sandra Foschi.

Notes from John Juhl, D.O., on Osteopathy and Prolotherapy

Doctors of osteopathy treat the whole person, not just the symptoms, by combining unique osteopathic principles with traditional diagnostic and therapeutic procedures to offer a balanced system of medical care. Osteopathy has traditionally focused on enhancing the body's ability to heal itself; however, osteopathic physicians may use all accepted medical means, including surgery, drugs, patient education, and manipulation of the body.

Most people come to an osteopath because they're having musculo-skeletal problems and are looking for a solution that does not involve surgery. One treatment they may receive from an osteopath is prolotherapy (short for proliferative injection therapy), which can be used to treat various types of pain, including arthritis; back pain; neck pain; fibromyalgia; sports injuries; whiplash; carpal tunnel syndrome; chronic tendinitis; torn tendons, ligaments, and cartilage; degenerated or herniated discs; TMJ (temporomandibular joint) pain; and sciatica. Prolotherapy uses a sugar-based solution that is injected into a ligament or tendon where it attaches to the bone.

This causes a localized inflammation in this weak area, which then increases the blood supply and flow of nutrients and stimulates the tissue to repair itself.

People often ask me what they should do to avoid the kinds of problems they want me to treat. The first answer is "Don't get old." The second answer is "Stay active." A study reported in the *Los Angeles Times* (D. R. Bassett et al., "Physical Activity in Old Order Amish Community," *Medicine & Science in Sports and Exercise* January 12, 2004) focused on the general health and obesity levels of ninety-eight members of an Old Order Amish community in Ontario, Canada. Although the Amish ate a high-calorie diet that included meat, potatoes, gravy, eggs, and pancakes, they had an obesity rate of only 4 percent (as opposed to more than 31 percent of the general U.S. population). It turns out they could eat what they wanted because they spent at least twenty hours in vigorous activities every week (heavy lifting, shoveling, tossing bales of hay) and had more than forty hours a week of moderate exercise (gardening, feeding farm animals, doing laundry by hand).

Most Americans don't have that kind of lifestyle. Our idea of exercise is something we do for perhaps half an hour, three times a week. There's a huge difference between what humans have been doing for the past four million years and what we've been doing for the past 150 years. In the *Los Angeles Times* article cited above, Dr. David Heber, director of the UCLA Center for Human Nutrition, noted that our genes haven't caught up to our modern diets and lifestyles. He said, "Our genes are perfectly adapted to another lifestyle, because you need those fat calories to plow the back forty."

We are not active enough in the Western civilized world. As a result, our bones are less dense, less mineralized. We've become more reliant on medication to maintain their density. We don't have the lean muscle mass we should. We're softer and we carry more weight because of our sedentary lifestyle.

People often come to see me knowing that they need to be less bound to their computers, televisions, and desks, but because of their years of inactivity, they begin to experience muscular-skeletal problems as soon as they start to exercise, and they feel that they just can't win. That's where we can help relieve the pain and also help guide them to a realistic schedule of activity.

This is important because the human body really is designed to repair itself through activity.

Notes from Albert Garcia on Massage Therapy

Massage, one of the oldest, simplest forms of therapy, is a system of stroking, pressing, and kneading different areas of the body to relieve pain and to relax, stimulate, and tone the body. Many types of massage are meant to relax the body and work out everyday kinks and sore spots. Other kinds of massage are more focused on relieving pain from sudden onset or long-standing injuries. Here are some examples:

- *Electromagnetic Massage:* This involves the application of micro-magnets at the site that needs attention. The magnets are very small, but they deliver a big punch. The low-voltage magnets help to improve the area by reversing pain, enhancing the body's endorphins, and reducing muscle contraction. The result is a twofold effect: a release of endorphins (which reduces the pain and makes you feel better) and a jump start on tissue healing by recharging the body's bioelectric field (which decreases healing time). Magnetic treatments are noninvasive and nontoxic, which makes them ideal for gentle, gradual body rebalancing and healing. Research demonstrates that magnetic treatments have strong actions on arthritis and bones, particularly in the treatment and prevention of osteoporosis.
- *Hot Stone Therapy:* This involves the placement of heated basalt lava stones and other therapeutic rocks and crystals on the body. During this treatment, the therapist uses traditional strokes of Swedish massage while holding a heated stone. Heated stones may also be left on specific points along the spine or other points on the body to help improve the energy flow. Hot stone therapy is excellent for deep-tissue penetration and is the perfect treatment to loosen tight muscles, relieve stress, and ease tension.

- *Clay Heat Therapy:* This treatment is especially effective for people who are experiencing severe muscular pain and cannot tolerate being massaged at the site of the discomfort. Bentonite clay, encased in canvas, is heated and placed on the problem area to flush out the lactic, uric, and carbonic acids retained in the muscles that account for the aches and soreness in the body. The process helps saturate the muscle with a very deep heat that forces out the toxins and helps restore the muscle to functioning wellness.
- *Ice Pack Therapy:* This is used mainly to treat sudden acute pain, poor circulation, and inflammation. It relieves pain and stabilizes blood flow at the site of an injury to reduce internal bruising and swelling. It is the ideal treatment for sprains and sports injuries.

Notes from Dr. Daniel Fenster on Chiropractic Care

Chiropractic is about structure affecting function. A chiropractor deals with the structure of the body, with the alignment of the spine and how that might affect function. It might affect function through nerves or through muscles, or it might affect the biomechanical function, meaning how the spine itself functions as a unit, or as what we call a kinetic chain.

There are two major concerns about structure when we reach our fifties. First is posture. As we age, gravity exerts a natural pull. Remember, we're holding our posture day after day, month after month, year after year. Eventually gravity is going to win by pulling on that posture. So your head starts to come more forward. You begin to hunch, and your shoulders become rounded. Without some kind of intervention, your alignment is going to be affected.

You may not even realize that you are out of alignment. Instead, you start to focus on the resulting symptoms, which could range from pain in various parts of the body to loss of function. Many people with these symptoms rely on drugs on like Advil for relief, but they don't change the underlying cause. I say, let's try and do something that will actually produce a change. When my patients come to me with these symptoms, I tell them this: If you were to lie on the beach for two weeks and drink a few margaritas, your symptoms would probably disappear. You don't need me just to make you feel better. You need me to make you feel better and to actually produce a change in your alignment and your structure, which will have lasting benefits.

The second concern about aging is that our spinal disks naturally dehydrate over time. Therefore, we lose flexibility. By keeping the spine in its best alignment, the structure in its best condition, we can slow that process. What I do is put my hands on a person's back and push their bones into a better alignment. I'm stretching them. I might use traction to elongate their spine or to restore a normal curve. My goal is to help the disk rehydrate by giving it more space.

Most people come to see me because of pain, stiffness, and decreased flexibility. What I'd like them to come for is to optimize their health and maintain flexibility—to be more proactive and less reactive. It's not just people who are sedentary and overweight who need alignment. People who exercise regularly often tell me that they don't need chiropractic. However, as with everything in life, there's a negative aspect to exercise: it tends to wear out the joints. Take a tip from professional athletes. They get adjusted (the technical term for the manipulations we perform) frequently because it increases their function. They don't wait until they have a problem; they prefer to be proactive so they will have an edge over their opponents. They want to function at 100 percent, because to them the difference between 100 percent and 99 percent might mean a championship.

169

Notes from Sandra Foschi on Physical Therapy

Physical therapy is the use of exercises and physical activities to help condition muscles and restore strength and movement, usually after injury or surgery. In fact, most people don't go to a physical therapist unless they have an injury, soreness, or tendinitis. By that time, inflammation has usually set in and their joints are already swollen.

I think all of us, especially as we age, should see a physical therapist for an evaluation. It's important to have someone look at you from head to toe—at your posture, the length of your muscles, and your arches—and ask such questions as these: What could use strengthening? Is the left side of the body weaker than the right, or vice versa? Then the therapist can help you devise a routine to improve those things and prevent injuries during your workouts.

The real issue is this: As we age, certain joints of the body become more vulnerable than others. For example, women's hips are usually very well-protected joints because they have such great padding (which women may or may not like), but many people have problems with their knees, where the ligaments and tendons have much less padding. Also, many people put unnecessary strain on their joints with repetitive movements. For example, you might go to the gym to exercise and use the same machines and work the same muscles in the same way every time. In this case, even if you're making the effort to go to the gym, you're not actually strengthening the muscles. Then, as you get older and have less lean muscle tissue to support your bones and joints, you become much more prone to injury. Add that to the normal wear and tear and degradation of cartilage that begins by the age of twenty-five, and you're left with a body full of very vulnerable joints.

Many people equate a longer time spent on a machine with a better workout. That's a big mistake and a waste of time. You're much better off running on a treadmill for twenty focused minutes and following that by some interval training—alternating short, fast bursts of intensive exercise with slow, easy activity.

It's also very important to do strength training with some type of resistance exercise such as free weights or Pilates. Resistance strengthens a muscle by overloading and challenging it. You have to challenge your muscles by constantly upping the ante or changing the routine.

It's all about balance. We all strive to strike balance in our personal lives, and we should do the same with our bodies. We need to have all our systems in balance. Often we make the mistake of concentrating on what we already do well. People who are already flexible but not strong usually love to do stretching exercises. People who are strong but not flexible concentrate on becoming stronger. When we don't pay attention to our areas of weakness, we create imbalances—and imbalances cause problems.

Oz Wraps It Up

There's no reason to live with the pains of the aging body. An occasional twinge is to be expected, but if pain becomes chronic, you need to see your doctor or health-care professional. As discussed above, several techniques and treatments are available to keep your joints and muscles strong and flexible well into your later years.

TWELVE

LONGEVITY AND THE BRAIN

KEEPING MENTALLY YOUNG

SENIOR MOMENTS — EVERYONE over fifty has them. You put your keys down five minutes ago, and now they're gone, disappeared, misplaced; you spend the next fifteen minutes searching, only to find them in the glass dish in the hall where you always leave them. You get up from the couch and walk into the den to get . . . something, although you now have no idea what. You're telling your children a story about your oldest and dearest friend—someone whose face you can see clearly in your mind, someone you speak to on the phone at least once a week—whose name you cannot for the life of you remember right now.

Perhaps our greatest fear is that these senior moments will turn into senior hours, and then senior lives. We are frightened to face a future of mental obliteration. It's not just the loss of cognitive function that we dread; it's the loss of *ourselves*.

Many factors contribute to mental decline, from changes in hormone levels (specifically in neurotransmitters, as noted in chapter 9), to poor oxygenation of the brain caused by lack of physical exercise, to years of exposure to toxins such as tobacco, alcohol, and even prescription drugs.

For many years, scientists believed that we lost more and more brain cells as we got older. Now we know that although brain cells do die off all the time, the process does not accelerate with age. It turns out that even into our seventies, the brain produces new neurons. It's true that the hippocampus, the brain's "filing system" that sends new information to its appropriate sections for storage and later recall, shrinks with age. But the hippocampus seems to compensate for its diminishing size by working even harder than it did when we were younger. It may take the brain longer to retrieve the information it needs or wants because these processes do slow down, but the processes are not usually irreparably damaged.

Many people never slow down at all. Take, for example, poet Stanley Kunitz, who died at the age of one hundred in May 2006. He never stopped writing poems and reading to live audiences, and at the age of ninety-five he was named poet laureate of the United States. This is an example of healthy aging at its finest.

Later in this chapter we hear about longevity and the brain from Dr. Eric Braverman, author of *The Edge Effect* and director of The Place for Achieving Total Health (PATH Medical). But first, here are my own strategies for keeping your brain in the healthiest shape possible for as long as possible.

173

Seven Strategies for Staying Mentally Young

To keep your brain active and functioning well, you can take these seven important steps to preserve and improve your current state of brain efficiency:

1. *Follow the New 50 Fusion Food Plan*: A diet rich in omega-3 fatty acids, antioxidants, and phytochemicals has been shown to improve cognitive performance and reduce inflammation, a major source of cell damage. A diet that includes plenty of fish—salmon, sardines, halibut, tuna, mackerel, bass, swordfish, mahi-mahi, trout, crab, and shrimp—plus olive oil and certain nuts and seeds will provide you with omega-3, an extraordinarily healthful nutrient (among many other nutrients critical for brain health). But fish isn't the only

brain food. Also, be sure to include plenty of colorful fruits and vegetables, which contain the vitamins, minerals, and phytochemicals that maintain brain health and enhance mental performance.

2. *Use Nutraceuticals*: We now know that there are very specific nutraceuticals that support brain function. If you're not getting enough omega-3 fatty acids from your diet, for instance, you may want to help improve brain function with EPA and DHA, two components of fish oil that are critical to brain health and efficiency. Omega-3 fats, specifically DHA, are required for the maintenance of normal brain function, especially as you get older, to maintain proper memory and manage learning. You'll learn more about nutraceuticals in the next chapter, but the good news is that you can protect your brain by making some very simple adjustments to your diet—for example, by adding ingredients such as fish, olive oil, and especially blueberries. A recent study at Tufts University showed that laboratory rats, equivalent in age to humans sixty to sixty-five-years old, that were fed blueberry extract in amounts equal to what in human terms would be half a cup of blueberries per day, had improved balance and neuromotor functioning as well as improved learning and memory skills. The rats that ate the blueberries had much higher levels of dopamine in their brains than did other groups of rats.

3. *Exercise on a Regular Basis*: Many studies have shown that physical exercise is good not only for your body but for your brain as well. As you become more active, you increase your breathing and heart rate, so that more oxygen and blood flow to the brain. Studies have even shown that exercise actually increases the number of brain cells—and exercise doesn't have to be strenuous to be effective. It turns out that walking is especially good for you because it increases the circulation of blood, oxygen, and glucose to the brain (it's possible that this is why we have a natural instinct to take a walk when we have a difficult problem to solve).

A study of senior citizens who walk regularly, conducted by Kenneth B. Schechtman of the Washington University School of Medicine and published in the *Annals of Behavioral Medicine* in August 2001, showed that walking improved learning ability, concentration, and abstract reasoning—and also cut the risk of stroke by 57 percent—in people who walked as little as twenty minutes a day. Another study (Laura Jean Podewils and Eliseo Guallar et al., "Physical Activity, APOE Genotype, and Dementia Risk: Findings from the Cardiovascular Health Cognition Study," *American Journal of Epidemiology* April 2005) surveyed 3,375 men and women over the age of sixty-five from 1992 to 2000. All were free of dementia at the time the study began. Researchers found that people who engage in a variety of physical activities have a better chance of avoiding Alzheimer's disease as they get older. Those people who avoided dementia tended to engage in a wide variety of activities, not only those requiring the most physical exertion. Although there was no definitive explanation for this, researchers suggested that it was because the variety required more activity in more sections of the brain. One more interesting study (Eric B. Larsin and Li Wang, et al., "Exercise Is Associated with Reduced Risk for Incident Dementia among Persons 65 Years of Age and Older," *Annals of Internal Medicine* January 17, 2006), which followed 1,740 people over the age of sixty-five for more than six years, showed that "Persons who exercised three or more times per week were more likely to be dementia-free than those who exercised fewer than three times per week."

4. *Surround Yourself with an Enriched Environment*: Studies have shown that when older rats are placed in enriched environments (with toys and other animals), they solve mazes faster than do rats in an environment with no stimuli. In addition, a March 2005 study from the University of Chicago found that mice that lived with chew toys, running wheels, and tunnels, which helped keep their brains and bodies active, had lower levels of Alzheimer's-associated brain plaques and protein buildup than did mice that lived in less stimulating

175

surroundings. Studies have also found that learning new things throughout your life helps maintain brain efficiency. The old saying "You can't teach an old dog new tricks" may be true for canines, but it is apparently not true for humans. In fact, it seems that the more you learn, the better your ability to learn, whether you are learning a foreign language, mastering a musical instrument, attending college, writing professionally, doing crossword puzzles or Sudoku (a logic-based number-placement puzzle), or playing competitive card games or board games. Also, retirement may not be so good for you after all; people who keep working past the traditional retirement age tend to remain healthier as they get older.

5. *Maintain Social Connections*: Scientists are not exactly sure why social connections spur healthy aging, but they know it works. A study that followed adults in their seventies for seven years found that those who maintained satisfying social relationships remained more mentally alert over the course of the study and experienced less age-related mental decline than did people who were more isolated. There are some theories as to why this is so. One posits that men and women who live alone tend not to eat as well, which could obviously affect their health and well-being. Another theory is that having people around improves your mental well-being because you feel loved and cared for. Social connections also motivate you to get out of the house and get moving. Research has also shown that people who have a close network of friends whom they can count on to help them cope with illness and stress tend to live longer and stay healthier, both physically and mentally.

6. *Engage in the Pursuit of Happiness*: The pursuit of happiness is one of the unalienable rights enumerated in the Declaration of Independence. Turns out, it's part of healthy aging, too. Researchers at the University of California at San Diego examined five hundred Americans, age sixty to ninety-eight, who lived independently and

had dealt with cancer, heart disease, diabetes, mental health conditions, or a range of other problems. To their surprise, the researchers found that happiness in old age may have more to do with attitude than actual health. The participants rated their own degree of successful aging on a scale from 1 to 10, with 10 being best, and despite everything they had suffered, the average rating was 8.4. In fact, optimism and effective coping styles were found to be more important to healthy aging than traditional measures of health and wellness. The researchers found this study encouraging because it showed that the best predictors of successful aging are within our control. Much recent research on this topic indicates that it's possible to feel happier, be more satisfied, and remain engaged with life regardless of one's circumstances. What's important to understand is that happiness doesn't necessarily float in on the wings of a bluebird—it's the lifelong pursuit of happiness that keeps you healthier and living longer.

177

7. *Get Enough Sleep*: These days, it's hard to find anyone who feels he or she gets enough sleep. But if you want a functioning, healthy brain, you've got to find a way to get those z's. As we get older, our sleep patterns change. We have greater difficulty falling asleep and more trouble staying asleep. And it's a myth that we don't need as much sleep as we used to. We all need between seven and nine hours of sleep a night. Older people, however, spend less time in deep, dreamless sleep, and they often awaken several times each night. There are also changes in our circadian rhythms as we get older, so we tend to become sleepier in the early evening and wake up earlier in the morning.

You can take steps to get more sleep. Your bedroom should be your sanctuary, a place that insulates you against the stress and pressures of the rest of the world. Make sure your bedroom is completely dark. Don't watch television in bed. You might try using white noise machines that mimic natural sounds such as waterfalls, chirping birds, or even human heartbeats. Avoid stimulants such as caffein-ated beverages, and note that while drinking alcohol in the evening may help you fall asleep, it actually increases awakenings during the night. The best thing you can do, however, is to train yourself not to go over the day's events in your mind or anticipate the future when you lie down to sleep.

Notes from Dr. Eric Braverman on Longevity and the Brain

As I wrote in my book *The Edge Effect*, the human brain is both exceedingly complex and remarkably simple. It has the power to send energy along billions of connections, evoking a sense of self that is capable at one moment of admitting the beauty of a rainbow and at the next of flying into a murderous rage.

What most people don't realize is that when your body is not working properly, the first thing to consider is the brain. The brain, and the biochemicals that reside there, control the body's health. Every day millions of people are diagnosed with ailments ranging from headaches to insomnia, depression, obesity, heart disease, and even cancer without taking the brain into consideration. Yet, in all those cases, the brain plays a critical role. If your brain chemistry is unbalanced, your body will be unbalanced.

Of course, the brain is also the home of thought and memory. A normal brain processes a thought at a speed of 300 milliseconds, or about one third of a second. Your "brain speed" is the rate at which electrical signals are processed throughout your body. When your brain speed slows, the brain doesn't have time to connect new stimuli to previously stored information before the next batch of stimuli rolls in. You can't react to stimuli as fast as you used to. If your thinking slows down to 400 milliseconds, you can no longer process logical thought. The brain does slow down with age, and it usually happens around the age of forty, when you begin to lose seven to ten milliseconds of brain speed per decade. We have about one tenth of a second to lose brain function, and every disease, every head trauma, every illness can slow us down.

Fortunately, it is possible to prevent the impairment this slowdown might cause by learning to keep your brain in top condition.

One step you can take is to find out whether you have a neurotransmitter imbalance and, if so, restore the balance through proper diet and nutraceutical supplements. Once that balance is restored, you can begin to look at the big picture—the five biggest predictors of longevity in our society:

1. *Normal Weight*: Most people don't think of weight management in terms of brain chemistry, but your increase in weight may be due to a decrease in levels of the neurotransmitter dopamine. We all know the dangers of obesity, but the difficulty of losing weight has not yet been successfully addressed by any scientific or technological advancements. The long-term answers may lie in normalizing the metabolism of the brain.

2. *Normal Behavioral Patterns*: We are a culture that is easily addicted to food, sex, television, alcohol, and recreational drugs—you name it, someone can become addicted to it. If you are prone to any of these extreme behaviors, you're probably damaging your health and your metabolism. Addictive behavior can be caused by a variety of factors, including brain chemistry, and it needs to be guarded very carefully if you are to live a long and healthy life.

3. *Getting Enough Sleep*: This point can't be overstated: Insufficient sleep affects your metabolism and can cause you to gain weight. It can cause depression. It weakens your immune system. Every night when you go to sleep, you shut off the central computer of your life and reboot it while you sleep. The computer dumps memory and throws things in the recycle bin, unloads saved documents, and restructures useful ones. Memories are consolidated. We know for a fact that the longest you can stay awake without getting psychotic is three days. The minimum amount of sleep you need is seven hours a night. The longer you go

179

without sleep, the more damage you cause to your brain chemistry and, therefore, your overall health.

4. *Controlling Anxiety, Depression, and Major Health Issues*: Brain breakdowns can wear out your life.

5. *Using Your Brain*: As stated earlier, an important aspect of longevity is keeping an active mental life to prevent cognitive decline.

Oz Wraps It Up

Although we have not yet learned to conquer diseases such as Alzheimer's that affect the brain, we are learning ways to halt the brain's decline. We are still in the early stages of discovering how the brain functions and how we can help it work better. The good news is that for most of us, senior moments will remain just that—transitory lapses that are basically harmless and usually become fodder for the funny stories we tell each other about the miseries of aging. The even better news is that science is steadily making new discoveries about what happens to the brain as it ages and about steps we can take to make sure we remain vital, healthy, and mentally alert throughout all our older years.

THIRTEEN

OZ'S GUIDE TO SUPPLEMENTS

THE NEW NUTRACEUTICALS

IF WE ALL ate as well as we should and exercised as much as we should, and if our bodies didn't change as we grew older, perhaps we wouldn't need to take any supplements (or nutraceuticals, as I prefer to call them). But we don't always eat as we should—Americans rarely get enough fruits and vegetables in their diets. We exercise when we can. And there's not much we can do about the changes that occur in our bodies over time. Even the healthiest among us have limits set by age, genetics, and circumstances.

That being said, we are fortunate in this day and age that many categories of supplements are available for enhancing and improving our bodies' natural abilities. As we get older our bodies need the support that nutraceuticals can supply for increased energy, clearer thinking, stronger bones, balanced moods, and enhanced immune systems.

Of course, not all nutraceuticals are covered here—that would be a book unto itself. The following list includes the supplements we believe are best designed to keep your body working in top form and to slow down the aging process. We don't expect you to take all of them; in fact, we don't want you to take all of them. You never want to overmedicate yourself, either with prescription drugs or vitamins. Read through the various descriptions, note which products you think will be helpful to you, and then discuss them with your health-care provider or nutritionist, especially if you are taking prescription or over-the-counter medications.

Nutraceuticals for Energy Production

ENADAlert (by Source Naturals)

ENADAlert is the trademarked name for NADH, which is the coenzyme form of vitamin B$_3$ (niacin). NADH is a naturally occurring nutrient for people desiring a stimulant-free energy boost. Quick-acting ENADAlert helps relieve drowsiness, restores alertness and energy, and boosts stamina and endurance. NADH is an energy-rich coenzyme that is essential for the production of ATP (adenosine triphosphate), the primary energy carrier in our cells. It is a central component in the energy-producing mechanism in our cells, and it is used in glycolysis, the first stage of the process in which the body breaks down glucose to use for energy. The brain, a highly energy-demanding organ, uses more glucose than any other organ. The brain, nerves, muscles, and heart require a constant supply of ATP energy in order to function. ENADAlert is one of the most powerful products with the most uniform impact on energy. It is also a mood lifter.

ProEndorphin (by Nutraceutics)

ProEndorphin is an effervescent energy cocktail designed to deliver energy in minutes. With a combination of B vitamins and amino acids, ProEndorphin supplies you with energy, endurance, and stamina. ProEndorphin is beneficial before, during, or after your workout or competition. Most people take ProEndorphin fifteen to thirty minutes before training or competition to boost their performance and energy levels, while others drink it during workouts to sustain endurance. Niacin is a B vitamin and a key ingredient in ProEndorphin. One quality of niacin is that it dilates blood vessels, creating a sensation of warmth that is often called the niacin flush. The reaction is usually mild, lasts five to fifteen minutes, and will disappear with continued use of ProEndorphin. ProEndorphin does not contain any added caffeine or synthetic stimulants. Kola nut, one of the ingredients in ProEndorphin, is derived from the seeds of the kola tree, which contain a small amount of naturally occurring caffeine. Kola nut has been traditionally used to combat physical and mental fatigue.

Vivaxyl (by Nutraceutics)

Vivaxyl takes your mental energy and physical staying power to new heights with nutrients that act quickly to jump-start your workouts, sex life, or lackluster days. Vivaxyl contains ginseng, B vitamins, and DL phenylalanine. Each serving also contains 2,800 milligrams of L-arginine, which is recognized for its benefits to sexual health.

183

EndFatigue Energy Revitalization Powder (by PhytoPharmica)

This powdered drink contains more than fifty vitamins, minerals, and other nutrients for exceptional health and sustained energy, including choline to help maintain mental alertness when you feel fatigue, as well as the vitamin B complex necessary for the healthy function of blood, brain, and nerve cells.

Nutraceuticals for Strong Bones

Oz Collagen/Hyaluronic Acid Powdered Drink

This product contains several important nutrients, including dietary collagen, hyaluronic acid, chondroitin, and vitamin C. It's especially good for aging joints, ligaments, and bones. One teaspoon twice a day mixed with water makes a powerful shake.

MSM *(by TriMedica)*

MSM is an abbreviation of methylsulfonylmethane, a form of sulfur that is found naturally in fresh fruits, vegetables, and many other foods. Unfortunately, food processing and soil depletion have dramatically decreased our supply of dietary sulfur. Sulfur is a fundamental building material of our bodies and is essential to our survival. It is often referred to as the beauty mineral because it softens tissue and keeps cells from becoming rigid. Without enough sulfur, cells become thin and tough, trapping in toxins and keeping out oxygen and nutrients. Sulfur is used by the body to form crucial proteins and amino acids.

MSM has an incredibly wide array of benefits, including these:

- Increased oxygenation, resulting in higher energy and better detoxification
- Improved skin, hair, and nails
- Increased blood circulation
- Reduced joint pain and stiffness
- Reduced inflammation
- Relief from asthma
- Increased mental alertness
- Controlled acidity in stomach and ulcers
- Rehabilitated intestinal tract lining
- Improved digestion and absorption of nutrients

Silica Gel *(by Body Essential)*

Silica has long been around as a supplement recommended for healthy hair. It is essential for maintaining healthy bones, nails, skin, and teeth. Collagen, tooth enamel, and even the gums benefit from bioavailable silica. It is found primarily in nature in a plant called horsetail. Use silica gel in combination with MSM for at least three months to see great improvement in the quality of your hair, skin, and nails.

For Women Only Hydroxyapatite (by AllergyResearchGroup)

This is a state-of-the-art bone-support formula containing hydroxyapatite, a form of calcium that is particularly well absorbed. It is formulated with a broad spectrum of nutrients and herbs that support the production of healthy bone tissue, including vitamins C, D, K, and B_6; folic acid; calcium; magnesium; zinc; and copper.

Nutraceuticals for Brain Power

Vinpocetine (by Pure Encapsulations)

This powerful memory enhancer has been used in Europe for many years. It facilitates cerebral metabolism by improving microcirculation (blood flow), stepping up brain cell production of ATP (the energy molecule), and increasing utilization of glucose and oxygen. This potent cognitive enhancer is used by doctors to treat acute stroke, inner-ear problems, and even headaches. Vinpocetine may also support oxygen release from hemoglobin, providing cells easier access to the oxygen they need. Furthermore, studies have reported that Vinpocetine may provide neuroprotection via its antioxidant properties.

Acetyl-L-Carnitine Arginate (by Life Extension)

Acetyl-L-carnitine (ALC) is an amino acid that maintains the cell's energy and has been shown to protect the brain against age-related degeneration and to improve memory, cognition, and mood. This product is effective even by itself (but don't take this product if you have epilepsy, because if you suffer from that disease, you're already too sensitive to neural stimulation). Acetyl-L-carnitine also protects against the buildup in the brain of lipofuscion, a fatty acid that deposits in the nerve cells and is associated with a reduction of cognitive powers. Acetyl-L-carnitine arginate is a novel molecular combination of the amino acids acetyl-L-carnitine and L-arginine. L-arginine is utilized to produce nitric oxide by the action of the enzyme tetrahydrobiopterin (THBP). L-arginine is a semi-essential amino acid synthesized by the body from ornithine. Arginine is important in bioenergetics because it is used by the body to produce creatine, the fuel source for ATP.

MaxiLIFE Choline Cocktail II (by Twinlab)

Choline Cocktail II is a scientifically advanced nutraceutical drink designed to increase mental alertness and energy. This quick-acting, easy-to-digest, brain-boosting formula contains a concentrated source of ginkgo biloba extract and guarana extracts, synergistically combined high potencies of cholineplus, citicholine, phosphatidylserine, DMAE, acetyl-L-carnitine, huperzine A, antioxidants, and other brain-boosting nutrients. MaxiLIFE Choline Cocktail II contains the most important nutrients and potencies for optimal brain function and is easier to consume on a daily basis than handfuls of tablets or capsules.

This tasty powder makes a good substitute for coffee and is an essential pick-me-up that helps nourish the brain and protect it from the wear and tear of aging. It even acts as a good hangover helper.

BrainWave Plus (by AllergyResearchGroup)

BrainWave Plus, a balanced formula of "smart nutrients" designed to enhance mental faculties, is based on the most current research of the underlying mechanisms of neurocognitive supportive nutrients. BrainWave Plus contains nutrients that collectively support a variety of mental functions, including blood circulation and neurotransmitter activity and production, which in turn support mental alertness, mood improvement, memory, and learning, to name a few. The latest additions to BrainWave Plus include huperzine A (*Huperzia seratta*), a traditional Chinese herb (Chien Tseng Ta) that is said to have significant beneficial effects on quality of life and memory retrieval for the patients involved in the study who had previously been experiencing various memory disorders; CDP-choline (cytidine 5-diphosphocholine), which quickly crosses the blood-brain barrier, increasing levels of neurotransmitters, enhancing cerebral energy metabolism, and activating the synthesis of critical components of cell membranes; and vinpocetine, an extract of periwinkle, which supports memory function by increasing circulation in the brain and increasing the rate at which brain cells produce ATP.

Nutraceuticals for Mood Enhancement

Pregnenolone (by Life Enhancement)

Pregnenolone is a hormone precursor that the body normally manufactures from cholesterol. Called the mother hormone, pregnenolone converts into other hormones, including DHEA (dehydroepiandrosterone), estrogen, testosterone, and progesterone. As with the steroid-hormone precursor DHEA, pregnenolone levels decline with age. When maintained and restored to youthful levels, pregnenolone helps to maintain memory and immune functions and may be an important step in the treatment of aging and the symptoms of aging. (Other hormones that decline with age and can be replaced include DHEA, melatonin, and the sex hormones testosterone, progesterone, and estrogen.)

Vinpocetine (by Pure Encapsulations)

In addition to enhancing brain power (see page 188), this nutraceutical is sometimes used as a mood enhancer.

Hyperimed St. John's Wort (by PhytoPharmica)

Dozens of controlled clinical trials have demonstrated that St. John's wort is effective as a mood stabilizer. It is also known to alleviate symptoms of mild to moderate depression and to improve stress tolerance, overall mental performance, and immune function. St John's wort has also been found to help control food cravings, improve energy, and dispel those annoying "winter blues."

Caution: Don't take St. John's wort if you are taking antidepressant monoamine oxidase inhibitors (MAOIs) such as Marplan or Nardil, or selective serotonin reuptake inhibitors (SSRIs) such as Prozac, Paxil, or Zoloft.

SAMe (by Jarrow Formulas)

SAMe (S-adenosylmethionine) is an amino acid derivative normally found in the body. It has been used as an antidepressant in Europe for years. A recent study from the University of Rome showed that SAMe is as effective as some conventional antidepressants. It has almost no side effects (although it should not be taken in combination with other antidepressants) and is believed to be one of the safest, most effective antidepressants in the world. It is also thought to offer significant support for liver function, and it has been found to protect against osteoarthritis and heart disease.

Nutraceuticals for Vision

For Your Eyes Only (by Roex)

For Your Eyes Only is a comprehensive formula of elements specifically combined to improved eye health. In addition to vitamins A, C, and E and the minerals copper, zinc, and selenium, which support the structure and function of the eye, For Your Eyes Only contains bilberry, which is rich in flavonoids, carotene, and anthrocyanosides, which help fortify vascular activity and deter arterial weakness. It is particularly effective for strengthening the eyes and vision because it contains lutein, a potent antioxidant carotenoid that helps protect the retina from damage caused by light or oxidation; pomegranate seed extract, which is proving to be a very powerful antioxidant in helping prevent pathological changes by free radicals to the lens of the eye; and curcumin, which also helps deter free radical damage and protects against exposure to ultraviolet light.

Super Zeaxanthin with Lutein (by Life Extension)

The carotenoids zeaxanthin and lutein, found in the macular region of the eye, help shield eyes from sun rays, computer screens, and other harmful forms of light that over time can cause photo-oxidative damage to the eyes. These fat-soluble antioxidants are uniquely able to absorb the most damaging portions of the light spectrum, helping to protect the lens, retina, and macula. In fact, zeaxanthin and lutein have been called conditionally essential nutrients because of their critical protective functions in the eye. With advancing age, however, concentrations of these precious carotenoids decline, leaving the eyes susceptible to health-related problems. While zeaxanthin is found in fruits and vegetables such as corn, peaches, and peppers, and lutein in green leafy vegetables such as spinach, most adults do not consume sufficient quantities of these foods to derive the carotenoids needed for optimal eye health. Super Zeaxanthin with Lutein provides standardized doses of these two critical nutrients, helping preserve the macular pigment density that is essential to healthy vision.

189

Nutraceuticals for Cleansing and Detoxification

Recancostat Powder (by Integrative Therapeutics)

Recancostat Powder is a patented oral supplement designed to boost the immune system. Combining the essential tripeptide glutathione and the important amino acid L-cysteine with a group of powerful antioxidants called anthocyanins, this supplement supports the immune system in both healthy individuals and those with varying degrees of compromised immunity. In addition, glutathione bolsters the structure of body proteins and assists in the transport of amino acids across cell membranes. Glutathione also helps the liver detoxify chemicals such as acetaminophen (the active ingredient in pain relief medication), copper, and cadmium.

Milk Thistle (by American Nutrition)

Milk thistle *(Silybum marianum)* contains a group of compounds known collectively as silymarin. Studies have shown silymarin to be one of the most effective liver-protective substances known to science. Silymarin is a potent antioxidant, ten times stronger than vitamin E. It has shown positive effects in treating nearly every known form of liver disease, including cirrhosis, hepatitis, necroses, and liver damage due to drug and alcohol abuse. The effectiveness of milk thistle is due to its ability to inhibit the factors responsible for liver damage, coupled with the fact that it stimulates production of new liver cells to replace old damaged cells. Milk thistle/silymarin also helps protect the liver from free radicals by stimulating the production of glutathione. Glutathione forms the basic foundation for building several powerful antioxidant enzymes. Like vitamin E and silymarin itself, these enzymes convert highly toxic free radicals into harmless compounds.

UltraClear Shake (by Metagenics)

UltraClear is a patented medical food specifically designed for the nutritional support of detoxification. No other medical product on the market has been patented for this use. This product is a powdered beverage drink mix that contains specific amounts and types of proteins, carbohydrates, and fats, that are easily absorbed and utilized. A specific core of nutrients and phytonutrients is added to help nutritionally support important detoxification activities. UltraClear assists with the removal of potentially harmful toxins associated with health conditions such as these:

- Alcohol/chemical dependency
- Chronic fatigue syndrome
- Fibromyalgia
- Generalized arthralgias
- Chemical sensitivity
- Atopic disorders
- Food allergies
- Migraine headaches

UntraClear is rich in the antioxidant vitamins A, C, E, and beta-carotene, which may help protect against free radicals generated during the detoxification process. This product not only offers the benefits of a detoxifying cleanser but can also be used as a full meal replacement.

OzClear Plus (by Xymogen)

191

OzClear Plus is a pleasant-tasting, rice protein–based, functional food meant to provide optimal cleansing nutrition for anyone suffering from conditions and symptoms associated with toxicity. OzClear Plus features a unique rice protein concentrate produced by a patented process that has a lower allergy potential than normal rice. This rice is fortified with the amino acids lysine and threonine, resulting in a complete, high-quality, easily digested vegetable protein.

Nutraceuticals to Support the Immune System

Folic Acid (by various manufacturers)

Folic acid is a B vitamin that is necessary for proper cell growth. If taken before and during early pregnancy from a multivitamin or fortified foods, folic acid can prevent 50 to 70 percent of some forms of birth defects, called neural tube defects, including spina bifida and anencephaly. Additional health benefits associated with folic acid include reductions in cardiovascular disease and in colon, cervical, and breast cancers. Studies have shown that folic acid, in combination with vitamins B_{12} and B_6, can help prevent recurrence of blocked arteries in patients who have undergone angioplasty, a procedure to unblock an artery of the heart. Folic acid may also help prevent Alzheimer's disease by protecting the neurons critical for learning and memory. Emerging research suggests that folic acid deficiency can also increase the brain's susceptibility to Parkinson's disease.

Probiotics (by various manufacturers)

The word "probiotic" means "for life" (as opposed to "antibiotic"). Probiotics are supplements containing the beneficial bacteria found in the human digestive tract that promote good gut health. For centuries, folklore has suggested that fermented dairy products containing live active cultures are healthful. Recent controlled scientific investigation supports these traditional views, suggesting that probiotics are a valuable part of a healthy diet. Probiotics enhance the immune system by preventing unfriendly organisms from gaining a foothold in the body. They prevent the overgrowth of yeast and fungus and produce substances that can lower cholesterol. Probiotics are widely recommended for the treatment and prevention of the fungal infection candidiasis, thrush, vaginal yeast infections, and athlete's foot. The benefits of probiotics include

- Inhibiting the growth of harmful bacteria that cause digestive stress
- Improving digestion of food and absorption of vitamins
- Stimulating the immune system, the body's natural defense mechanism
- Helping make vitamins that are needed by the body

Aloe C Defense (by Nutraceutics)

Aloe C Defense is made from the purest form of natural whole aloe vera, named beta-mannin, containing a highly potent complex of polysaccharides, enzymes, amino acids, vitamins, and minerals like sulfur, iron, calcium, copper, potassium, and more that may help you overcome feelings of fatigue and stress. The aloe vera is freeze-dried immediately after harvesting to preserve its bioactivity. In addition to providing 1,000 milligrams of vitamin C per tablet, once activated, this natural energy cocktail energizes your immune system, supplies you with a powerful antioxidant, and is a great way to start your day or boost you along the way. Vitamin C is a wonder vitamin and is essential to everything from the production of collagen (the tissue that holds us together) to reducing the inflammatory eicosanoids that damage our bodies.

Coenzyme Q10 (by Life Extension)

The mitochondria are the cell's energy powerhouses, and coenzyme Q10 (CoQ10) is an essential component of healthy mitochondrial function. CoQ10 is required to convert fats and sugars into cellular energy; yet the natural production of CoQ10 declines precipitously with advancing age. When the body has an ample amount of CoQ10, the mitochondria can work most efficiently throughout the entire body, in cells everywhere, including the most densely populated area—the heart.

Cruciferous Vegetable Extract Capsules (by Life Extension)

Scientists have identified specific extracts from cruciferous vegetables (*e.g.,* broccoli, cauliflower, Brussels sprouts) that modulate hormones in a way that helps maintain healthy cell division. For instance, animal studies have shown that the cruciferous vegetable extract indole-3-carbinol (I3C) modulates estrogen hormones by favorably changing the ratio of protective 2-hydroxyestrone versus the damaging 16-hydroxyestrone. This is a unique protective dietary supplement with the full-spectrum benefits of fresh vegetables.

Pomegreat Pomegranate Juice Concentrate (by Jarrow Formulas)

The pomegranate *(Punica granatum)* has long been recognized as a fruit with many health benefits. The pomegranate tops all other conventional fruits, including blueberries and strawberries, in its ORAC (oxygen radical absorbance capacity) value, which ranks it as one of the most powerful antioxidant fruits. Pomegranate juice contains a wide range of polyphenolic compounds—including ellagic and gallic acid, anthocyanins and tannins, and especially punicalagin, a powerful antioxidant—that protect cardiovascular function and accurate cellular replication. Pomegranate juice has these properties:

- Decreases low-density lipoprotein (LDL) oxidation
- Enhances cellular (macrophage) glutathione
- Helps maintain regular platelet activity
- Reduces the activity of angiotensin converting enzyme (ACE) and supports normal vascular contraction
- Promotes normal cell function and replication

Caution: People who take hypertensive medications should monitor their blood pressure closely when taking pomegranate juice. Those who are allergic to many plants should consult a physician before taking pomegranate or pomegranate products.

Green Tea (by various manufacturers)

Green tea, which originated in China four hundred years ago, has been used for centuries to treat everything from headaches to depression. It may help protect against cancer and heart disease, and it may also help strengthen the bones in postmenopausal women. Research also indicates that drinking green tea lowers total cholesterol levels and improves the ratio of good (HDL) cholesterol to bad (LDL) cholesterol. Here are some of the medical conditions for which drinking green tea is reputed to be helpful:

- Cancer
- Rheumatoid arthritis
- High cholesterol levels
- Cardiovascular disease
- Infection
- Impaired immune function

Studies also show that green tea may keep your teeth healthy by reducing the amount of plaque-causing bacteria in your mouth, apparently because of the presence of polyphenols, which seem to inhibit the formation of bacteria that promote cavities.

195

IGG 2000 (by Xymogen)

IGG 2000 represents a breakthrough in immunoglobulin supplementation. It is a highly concentrated, nondairy source of serum-derived immunoglobulin antibodies and immunoproteins. It possesses three times more IGG (gamma-immunoglobulin) and total immunoglobulins than colostrum and has twice as much cysteine, an important amino acid for maintaining glutathione levels.

Nutraceutical Antioxidants

OZ Longevity Pak (by Oz Garcia)

Developed with some of the top scientists in the antiaging field, the OZ Longevity Pak includes the latest scientific nutritional breakthroughs to promote youthful health for optimal results. It contains powerful nutraceuticals designed to

- Support youthful-looking skin
- Support healthy brain power and performance
- Help defend against the ravages of stress
- Support healthy blood circulation and heart health
- Promote healthy hormonal function
- Add vigor and vitality when combined with healthy diet and exercise

OZ Longevity Pak has been enhanced with lutein, lycopene, vinpocetine, green tea, and grape seed extracts as well as a proprietary blend of CoQ10. The content of our essential fatty acid formula has been boosted to 1,200 milligrams. These advanced improvements are unparalleled in the field today.

196

Maxogenol (by Nutraceutics)

Maxogenol contains grape seeds, grape skins, blueberries, and red grapes. Modern science has discovered that dark-colored berries and red and blue grapes contain a virtual treasure trove of health-preserving, possibly even life-extending, ingredients. This product is good for everyone, including children and even pets. It also contains green tea for maximum antioxidant protection.

Vitamin E Alpha-Tocopherol (by various manufacturers)

A large prevention trial conducted by the National Cancer Institute and the National Public Health Institute of Finland, consisting of 29,133 male smokers (as reported in the *Journal of the National Cancer Institute*, March 18, 1998), showed that men fifty to sixty-nine years old who took 50 milligrams of alpha-tocopherol (a form of vitamin E) daily for five to eight years had 32 percent fewer diagnoses of prostate cancer and 41 percent fewer prostate cancer deaths than did men who did not receive vitamin E.

Additional benefits of vitamin E have been exhaustively documented, from reducing the risk of Alzheimer's disease to lowering the risk of coronary heart disease, preventing blood clotting, and reducing the risk of certain cancers.

Another age-related problem is deteriorating vision. A study was conducted by the Johns Hopkins University School of Hygiene and Public Health (Päivi Rouhiainen, Harri Rouhiainen, and Jukka T. Salonen, "Association between Low Plasma Vitamin E Concentration and Progression of Early Cortical Lens Opacities," *American Journal of Epidemiology* 144, 1996: 496–500) to determine the association between blood levels of vitamin E and the development of cataracts. The study looked at 410 men over the course of three years and concluded that the men with the lowest levels of vitamin E had a 3.7 times greater risk of cataract formation than did those with the highest levels of vitamin E.

Note: You want not just any vitamin E but a combination that includes d-gamma-tocopherol and d-alpha tocopherol, which are two extremely bioactive forms of vitamin E and should constitute part of a well-designed supplement program.

197

Life Extension Mix (by Life Extension)

Life Extension Mix contains ninety-two unique vegetable, fruit, and herbal extracts; amino acids; vitamins; minerals; and special antioxidants. The Life Extension Mix formula is fortified with botanical extracts that help maintain health. This product is the "Swiss army knife" of nutraceuticals, containing ninety-two super-high-potency ingredients that target everything from inhibiting glycosylation to improving microcapillary circulation.

Resveratrol Caps (by Life Extension)

Findings from published scientific literature indicate that resveratrol may be the most effective plant extract for maintaining optimal health. Red wine contains resveratrol, but the quantity varies depending on where the grapes are grown, the time of harvest, and other factors. After years of relentless research, a standardized resveratrol extract is now available as a dietary supplement. This whole-grape extract contains a spectrum of polyphenols that are naturally contained in red wine, such as proanthocyandins, anthocyanins, and flavonoids. The resveratrol used in these products is extracted from organic grapes.

Blueberry Capsules (by Life Extension)

According to a 2004 study (X. Wu and G. R. Beecher, et al., "Lipophilic and Hydrophilic Antioxidant Capacities of Common Foods in the United States," *Journal of Agriculture and Food Chemistry* 52, June 16, 2004), when researchers analyzed fruits and vegetables for their antioxidant capability, blueberries came out on top, rating highest in their capacity to destroy free radicals. Scientists have recently discovered mechanisms to explain how blueberries can improve memory and restore healthy neuronal function to aging brains. Blueberry extracts help maintain healthy blood flow via several mechanisms, including healthy LDL oxidation, normal platelet aggregation, and maintenance of endothelial function. When blood flow is interrupted to the brain (ischemia), significant and permanent damage often results. In rats that were fed blueberries, the area of their brains damaged by ischemia was 50 percent smaller than that in the control rats. One of the active constituents found in blueberries is anthocyanins; blueberry anthocyanins are considered nature's most potent antioxidants.

Recancostat Powder

See page 189, under "Nutraceuticals for Cleansing and Detoxification."

For Your Eyes Only

See page 188, under "Nutraceuticals for Vision."

Nutraceuticals for Skin and Hair

Silica

See page 183, under "Nutraceuticals for Strong Bones."

199

MSM (by TriMedica)

See page 183, under "Nutraceuticals for Strong Bones."

L-Cysteine (by Twinlab)

L-cysteine serves as a precursor for the synthesis of proteins, glutathione, taurine, coenzyme A, and inorganic sulfate. It is a nonessential amino acid that is an important component of hair, nails, and the keratin of the skin. L-cysteine stabilizes the protein structure and aids in the formation of collagen, thereby promoting healthy skin, hair, and nail texture. It is also used in the treatment of respiratory disorders such as chronic bronchitis, helps decrease recovery time from surgical operations and burns, and stimulates white blood cell activity in the immune system to help build resistance to disease.

Alpha-Lipoic Acid (by Xymogen)

Alpha-lipoic acid (ALA) is considered the universal antioxidant. It boosts levels of glutathione in all cells, exhibits antioxidant activity in almost all tissues of the body, and improves the antioxidant functionality of vitamin C, vitamin E, and Coenzyme Q10. It reduces inflammation, pumps up the immune system, and helps the human body knit together tissue injuries. Alpha-lipoic acid is known to fight free radicals in any part of the cell and even in the spaces between them. It also signals tissue-repairing compounds, including one called transcription factor AP-1, to begin working. Alpha-lipoic acid allows AP-1 to "digest" damaged collagen, resulting in the elimination and erasure of wrinkles. Alpha-lipoic acid also appears to protect against glycation by blocking the attachment of sugar to protein. It may reverse glycation damage and protect collagen from the toxic effects of sugar.

Nutraceuticals with Essential Fatty Acids

Oz Ultra Pure Arctic Oil (by Xymogen)

Fish such as salmon, sardines, halibut, tuna, mackerel, bass, swordfish, mahi-mahi, cod, and trout, and shellfish such as crab and shrimp, are high in omega-3 fatty acids, as are olive oil, fish oil, and many nuts and seeds. Omega-3 fatty acids are the building blocks of the body's anti-inflammatory eicosanoids, the ones that control inflammatory damage to tissue.

Three major types of omega-3 fatty acids are ingested in foods and used by the body: alpha-linolenic acid (ALA), eicosapentaenoic acid (EPA), and docosahexaenoic acid (DHA). Once they have been eaten, the body converts ALA to EPA and DHA, the two types of omega-3 fatty acids more readily used by the body. Extensive research indicates that omega-3 fatty acids reduce inflammation and help prevent certain chronic diseases such as heart disease and arthritis. These essential fatty acids are highly concentrated in the brain and appear to be particularly important for cognitive and behavioral function. Recent evidence shows that a deficiency of DHA (a component of omega-3 fats) during pregnancy can impair a child's intelligence and visual acuity.

It is very important to maintain a balance between omega-3 and omega-6 fatty acids in a healthy diet, which should consist of roughly one to four times more omega-6 fatty acids than omega-3 fatty acids. The typical American diet tends to contain eleven to thirty times more omega-6 fatty acids than omega-3 fatty acids. Many researchers believe that this imbalance is a significant factor in the rising rate of inflammatory disorders in the United States. By following the New 50 Fusion Food Plan, you will consume a healthy balance between omega-3 and omega-6 fatty acids.

Flax Oil (by various manufacturers)

Like most vegetable oils, flax oil, also called flaxseed oil, contains linoleic acid, an essential fatty acid needed for survival. But unlike most oils, it also contains significant amounts of another essential fatty acid, ALA. Flaxseed oil may help lower cholesterol, and research indicates that it may also lower blood pressure. Flaxseed—the most concentrated vegetarian source of omega-3 fatty acids found in nature—contributes to heart and nerve health while providing an energy source for the body.

201

AN OLIVE A DAY?

 A study published in the January 2005 issue of the *Annals of Oncology* says that the oleic acid found in olives and olive oil can help prevent cancer, especially breast cancer: "Oleic acid, the main monounsaturated fatty acid of olive oil, suppresses Her-2/neu (erb B-2) expression and synergistically enhances the growth inhibitory effects of trastuzumab (Herceptin™) in breast cancer cells with Her-2/neu oncogene amplification." It seems that oleic acid suppresses the function of oncogenes, the genes that cause regular cells to mutate and grow into tumors. Dr. Javier Menendez of Northwestern University Feinberg School of Medicine, who headed the study, says that his team determined that the oleic acid blocks the action of Her-2/neu oncogene, found in about 30 percent of all breast cancer patients. The study also found that oleic acid improved the effectiveness of a popular breast cancer drug called Herceptin.

Coconut Oil (by various manufacturers)

Coconut oil is rich in lauric acid, which is known for being antiviral, antibacterial, and antifungal. Coconut oil is also used by people with thyroid problems to increase body metabolism and lose weight. Coconut oil is now being recognized by the medical community as a powerful tool against immune diseases. Several studies have been conducted on its effectiveness, and much research is currently being done on the incredible nutritional value of pure coconut oil.

Conjugated Linoleic Acid (by various manufacturers)

Conjugated linoleic acid (CLA) is a fatty acid found in foods and is a main component of red meat that may prevent cancer. Further research has shown that in addition to being a potent anticancer agent, it's also an anticatabolic agent (meaning that it protects against muscle loss), an immune stimulant, and, through a unique mechanism, a fat-burning agent. CLA has become a popular supplement among fitness enthusiasts because of this last feature. It also is a potent antioxidant that lowers cholesterol, and it may be useful in a wide range of inflammatory disorders because of its ability to reduce an inflammatory eicosanoid known as prostaglandin E_2 (PGE_2).

Mega-GLA (by Life Extension)

As people age, chronic systemic inflammation can inflict degenerative effects throughout the body. A primary cause of this destructive cascade is the production of cell-signaling chemicals known as inflammatory cytokines. Along with these dangerous cytokines, imbalances of hormonelike messengers called prostaglandins also contribute to chronic inflammatory processes. The body needs fatty acids to survive and is able to make all but two of them: linoleic acid in the omega-6 family and linolenic acid in the omega-3 family. These two fatty acids must be supplied by diet and are therefore considered essential fatty acids (EFAs). Omega-6 fatty acids are well supplied in meat and vegetable oils. However, not all omega-6 fatty acids are of equal value. Gamma-linolenic acid (GLA), found in evening primrose oil, borage oil, and black currant oil, is an important fatty acid that plays a beneficial role in healthy prostaglandin formation. There are "good" prostaglandins and "bad" prostaglandins. Too much of the wrong prostaglandins can produce inflammation—for instance, cramping during a menstrual period (that's why you take Motrin, which is a prostaglandin inhibitor). Black currant oil plays a role in the production of the healthy prostaglandins that work to control inflammation, pain, and discomfort.

This particular product includes sesame lignans. New information about the ability of sesame to prevent the conversion of GLA into arachidonic acid indicates that many more people may now be able to benefit from supplemental GLA.

Nutraceuticals for Hormones and Libido

ProEstron (by Nutraceutics)

ProEstron is an alternative way to help manage the symptoms of menopause, designed to address the specific needs of women over the age of forty. ProEstron is formulated to work with the natural rhythm of the female body to promote physical and emotional balance during perimenopause and menopause. Many women see improvements with their menopausal symptoms in as short a time as three to four weeks, although it may take four to twelve weeks to feel the full benefits of ProEstron.

NOW Cream (by Apothecure)

For those who wish to use enhancement products without a prescription, topical creams are a fantastic alternative. NOW (Natural Orgasms for Women) cream, a topically applied enhancement product that contains L-arginine, topical vasodilators such as niacin, oils, and several other ingredients, has yielded some amazing results. Women who have used this product report increased enjoyment during intercourse and orgasm. Application of the NOW cream can be used intravaginally via a vaginal applicator tube (about 0.5 to 1 gram)—which evidently stimulates the Graffenberg spot (G-spot)—or topically to the clitoris. Application should be completed thirty minutes to two hours before intercourse.

Big Blue Capsules (by OPCPure)

The key ingredient in this product, L-arginine, also called just arginine, has appeared in many products in the past couple of years, gaining popularity as a nonprescription treatment for high cholesterol and as an active ingredient in sexual-support products. It is used to release insulin in the pancreas, and it is a component of the human growth hormone in the pituitary gland. L-arginine is required for the body to synthesize nitric oxide, which enables the arterial system to retain its youthful elasticity. Nitric oxide also helps produce endothelial relaxation factor, which is needed by the arterial system to expand and contract with each heartbeat.

Nutraceuticals for Weight Loss

Conjugated Linoleic Acid (by various manufacturers)

See page 200, under "Nutraceuticals with Essential Fatty Acids."

CM3 Alginate (by Abnempillan & Co., imported from Germany)

The most sensible way of dealing with excess weight is to follow a low-calorie, low-fat diet. But diets often fail because hunger pangs make dieting an act of willpower. CM3 Alginate, a patented formulation based on brown seaweed *(Laminaria digitata),* can help you succeed by tricking your brain into thinking that you're full. CM3 Alginate dissolves in the stomach and expands into a soft, gel-like solid. The principle of action, based on pure physics, brings about a long-lasting feeling of satiation. CM3 Alginate makes it easier to eat less and to lose weight naturally.

Energenics (by Metagenics)

This is an extremely well-designed product for improving your resting metabolic rate, or the rate at which you burn calories at rest. This product is especially effective if you have low thyroid function, which can be determined by medical analysis. It's also good for helping an aging metabolism perform better.

ZyMelt (by Nutraceutics)

ZyMelt was designed to support efforts to lose weight and fat. It is a physique-enhancing, weight-loss supplement that benefits both men and women. Fors-Lean, a key ingredient in ZyMelt, is a standardized extract from the root of the *Coleus forskohlii* plant, a member of the mint family. *Coleus forskohlii* is the only known plant source of forskolin, a compound that may increase lean body mass and therefore optimize body composition. Forskolin facilitates a cascade of biochemical events in the body that allow fat cells to be used as energy, and it helps utilize hormones to maintain and/or increase lean body mass. Specifically, forskolin activates the main enzyme involved in the production of a metabolic molecule called cyclic adenosine monophosphate (cAMP), which is indispensable to many bodily functions—triggering metabolic processes and thermogenesis (the body's main fat-burning mechanism) as well as increasing muscle-building hormones.

Whey Protein Shakes (by various manufacturers)

Protein powders come in many variations. Some are egg-based, some are soy-based, and some (my favorites) are whey-based. Shakes are a great way to start most mornings. High-quality whey-based powders, besides providing the macronutrients for building muscle and body tissues, also deliver a vast array of immune support nutrients, such as naturally occurring immunoglobulins. They are high in protein value, low in carbohydrates and fats, and rich in antioxidants, especially those involved in liver detoxification. These shakes are highly functional foods that can be used as part of weight-loss or muscle-building programs as well as part of a general maintenance program.

EPILOGUE

LIFE LESSONS

I have a daughter who's twenty-six. If I want to look at a twenty-six-year-old, I'll look at her. I don't want to look twenty-six; I just really want to look great. But you want to look great and look as if you're normal. Once you start with surgery, you really do look different. And it doesn't necessarily look better. It becomes like an addiction, and I'd rather have staying healthy be my addiction. Do I look as if I'm twenty-six? No, but I look and feel terrific.

You have to have a good attitude about health but not be frantic if you have a "bad" meal or if you miss a day of exercise. And a lot of that franticness comes from being around other people who are frantic. You go to the gym and you find yourself in a room with a big mirror, and everyone is vying for the front spot to be near the instructor, and each person is comparing her body with everyone else's. Once you get into that, it's very hard not to become obsessed with it. So don't even start that way. Do things that are going to make you look great but that you can do your whole life.

A lot of it is just protecting yourself and knowing what works for you. You have to be careful about who you're with and who you choose to have as friends and who you choose to be your partner.

Most of the time, I don't worry about getting older. It does get to me when I see my parents getting older and they're getting fragile, and you realize that life goes by in a blink. That's when it's good to take stock and appreciate what you have and try and get the most out of each day. Believe me, I'm not like that every day, but it really is true. It all goes by so quickly that you just can't get hung up on every little thing. You've got to do the best you can and put some meaning into your life and appreciate what you have. We all get caught up in "stuff," but realize when you're getting caught up that you need to take a step back and say, "Wait a second—this isn't who I want to be, and this isn't the way I want to do it." And hopefully you'll take a deep breath and you'll be able to manage and not have it overwhelm you. Because we all get overwhelmed at times. But when you are overwhelmed, you just have to go on and do the best you can. You'll get through it in the end.

RICKI LUBART

This is how I feel about being fifty-one. I think it's an interesting evolution for me. I raised three children. I worked before I had them, and then I was a stay-at-home mom. I got totally bored with that. I saw that eventually they were going to leave, and I knew that I needed to have something to do for myself. That's when I started Paris Personal Shopper in 2001. It had to be something that was fun, something that I loved, and since my children were still at home, it had to be on a part-time basis. Later on, it was Oz who actually said, "You should write a book; it will change things." And it did.

I have reinvented myself at fifty. My life has changed. I feel great. Maybe I don't have as much energy as I did when I was twenty, but I'm wiser. Before I turned fifty, I had a voice in the fashion world, but it was a small voice. Now my voice is bigger and stronger and louder. Now people are finally hearing me. I feel that I'm being validated for all my hard work and the experience.

At fifty, I am recognized for what I know, and I feel really good about it. The chapter of raising kids is over. Now I have my work, which is very exciting. I feel that I'm a pioneer. There are so many opportunities, and the universe is open to me. As long as my skin is good, my body is good, and I still have the energy, whether I'm fifty-one or seventy-one or thirty-one, it doesn't matter. I'd rather be fifty-one than twenty-one, because I think that the experience is so valuable, and the knowledge and wisdom make up for it.

SUSAN TABAK

Of course getting older is on my mind, but it's nothing that I dwell on. It's nothing that depresses me. However, it puts life into a different perspective that I haven't had before. I have a greater realization of my finitude that I did not have when I was younger. And time passes so much more quickly each year. That's actually a gift, because you choose to let certain things go by the wayside; you have a clearer understanding of what's important to you and what's not.—and a greater freedom to let go of the things that are not.

Of course, if I had my druthers and I could put this head back on my body of thirty years ago . . . truthfully, though, I like who I am and who I've evolved into, and I wasn't this person thirty years ago. I'm very pragmatic. It is what it is. Am I going to beat my head against the wall? There's nothing I can do about getting older, so I do everything I can to increase the joy in my life. And I'm not going to be self-antagonistic about things that I have no control over. That's not how I want to spend my energy. Ten years from now, I might be looking back at this age, wishing I was in my fifties again. Why are we always looking back? Why don't we look in a different direction or have a different perspective? That's what I do. You have a choice here. One causes angst, and one doesn't. My choice is to go with less angst.

JAN HOERRNER

And Finally, Oz Wraps It All Up

My goal in writing this book was to give you options.

I knew from the very beginning that I couldn't expect anyone reading this book to undergo every lifestyle change and treatment presented here. I do expect that you will find several options throughout this book that are applicable to you in your life, and some methods that you can begin to incorporate immediately. In following the *Redesigning 50* program, your goal is to peel off a certain amount of wear and tear on your body—perhaps as much as ten to fifteen years—to make sure that you are as healthy and vital as you can possibly be, no matter what your chronological age.

I hope that you consider as many options as you can. There is no one route

How do I feel about getting older? There are parts of me that feel still very young. Sometimes I totally forget that I'm in my fifties. I look in the mirror and I don't know if it's my nutrition or if it's a combination of all the things I've done. But every once in a while people do think I'm in my thirties, and they really don't believe how old I am. Of course, there are some aches and pains. I'm not sure if the aches and pains are because I'm not being careful—maybe if I stopped drinking coffee and stopped eating ice cream, my aches and pains would magically go away. As human beings, we're constantly in the world and not necessarily eating perfectly all the time. How much can supplementation and diet and constantly monitoring and changing improve things? I'm not sure, but I do know that I've been through times where all of a sudden my allergies are out of control and I go back to healthier eating and better habits, and I feel well again.

My expectations for the next fifty years are pretty high. I see a lot of different research coming out of different universities. There are some new forms of resveratrol research coming out of Harvard that say it has the same effect as calorie restriction, which has a profound effect on the strength and vitality of your cells. I actually believe that a lot of these new discoveries are going to come to our rescue and make a difference in our health, and I want to be there when it happens. We have no idea what an eighty-year-old will look like thirty years from now. I'm excited about the future and looking forward to how far we can push the envelope.

JOHN ASLANIAN

to an antiaging lifestyle. There's no fixed road map to life extension. There are many ways to manage and regulate your body's efficiency. What you want to strive for is a synergistic lifestyle in which many elements come together and allow for the emergence of a stronger body and outlook.

For myself, I've completely redesigned what it means to be in my fifties, and I don't feel all that different from the way I did two decades ago. I use every possible option in the *Redesigning 50* program to my advantage. And I think the people we've interviewed for this book have shown that it's possible to take very practical approaches to regulating the aging process. We're not aging the way our parents did. With the few exceptions of those who were fortunate enough to have the genes for good health, our parents had difficult older years. They didn't understand how detoxification could make a difference in health. They didn't know the importance of exercise and fitness. They certainly didn't have the scientific breakthroughs to which we are privy.

I urge you to take advantage of what we now know and have available to us. If you incorporate small changes into your life, it won't take you long to see and feel the benefits. And you can start now. Walk just twenty minutes a day, and you can greatly reduce your risk of heart disease, cancer, and even Alzheimer's. Try a mini-cleanse and then maybe a longer one. Be careful about your food choices. Watch how you manage stress in your life. None of these things require tremendous effort; yet they are tremendously important.

If you follow just a small portion of the *Redesigning 50* program, you'll be amazed at how much better you'll look and feel. Now it's all up to you.

Please let me know how you're doing. Tell me what you tried and how it worked. Send me before-and-after photos. Ask me questions; I'll do my best to answer. You can contact me at

Oz Garcia
10 West 74th Street
New York, NY 10023
info@ozgarcia.com

And don't forget to visit my Web site: www.ozgarcia.com. I look forward to hearing from you.

RESOURCE GUIDE

Individuals and Organizations

Dr. Lisa Airan (cosmetic dermatologist)
910 5th Avenue
New York, NY 10021
212-400-0999
www.lisaairan.com

Maria Alonso (massage therapist)
201-618-0394
www.ukneadtherapy.com

David Barton (personal trainer, owner of
   David Barton Gyms)
DavidBartonGym
david.barton@dbgym.com
www.davidbartongym.com

Biophysical250
Biophysical Corp.
3300 Duval Road
Austin, TX 78759
512-623-4900
www.biophysicalcorp.com

Dr. Lionel Bissoon
   (mesotherapist)
Mesotherapy & Estetik
10 West 74th Street, Suite 1F
New York, NY 10023
212-579-9136
www.mesotherapy.com

David Bouley (chef)
Bouley
120 West Broadway
New York, NY 10013
212-964-2525
www.bouley.net

Dr. Eric Braverman (director of PATH
   Medical)
PATH Medical
185 Madison Avenue, 6th Floor
New York, NY 10016
212-213-6155
www.pathmed.com

Buchinger Clinic
Forstweg 39
D-31812 Bad Pyrmont, Germany
+49-5281-1660
Klinik.dr.ott@buchinger.de
www.buchinger.de

Gordon Chiu (beauty and skin
*   consultant)*
Gordon Yourself LLC
P. O. Box 616
Summit, NJ 07902
917-288-8817
www.gordonyourself.com

Robin Cofer (yoga and meditation
*   teacher)*
845 United Nations Plaza, 90th floor
New York, NY 10017
646-408-0511
212-758-8760
recofer@aol.com

Cornelia Spa
663 5th Avenue, 8th Floor
New York, NY 10022
212-871-3051 or 866-663-1700
www.cornelia.com

Daniel Davidson (geneticist)
M.D. Darwin Labs
P.O. Box 19077
Miami Beach, FL 33139

305-673-2526
www.MDDarwin.com

Bruce Dean (makeup artist)
646-271-6671
Brucedean01@yahoo.com
www.BruceDean.com

Dr. Roni DeLuz (founder of Martha's
*   Vineyard Diet Detox)*
Martha's Vineyard Holistic
    Retreat
Franklin Street
Vineyard Haven, MA 02568
508-693-0001 or 800-595-9996
www.mvdietdetox.com

Equinox
Suzanne Meth
smeth@equinoxfitness.com
www.equinoxfitness.com

Frédéric Fekkai (hairstylist)
New York Salon
Henri Bendel, 4th Floor
712 5th Avenue
New York, NY 10022
212-753-9500
Beverly Hills Salon
444 North Rodeo Drive
Beverly Hills, CA 90210
310-777-8700
www.fredericfekkai.com

Dr. Daniel Fenster
Complete Chiropractic Center
30 East 60th Street, Suite 302
New York, NY 10022
212 737-9000

Dr. Richard Firshein
Firshein Center for Comprehensive
Medicine
1230 Park Avenue
New York, NY 10128
212-860-0282

Sandra Foschi (physical therapist)
Health SOS
139 East 57th Street, 3rd Floor
New York, NY 10022
212-753-4767
Sandra@healthsos.com
www.healthsos.com

Albert Garcia (massage therapist)
Restore Spa
10 West 74th Street, Suite 1D
New York, NY 10023
212-877-5500
www.restorespa.com

The Golden Door Spa
P. O. Box 463077
Escondido, CA 92046
760-744-5777 or 800-424-0777
www.goldendoor.com

John Juhl, D.O. (osteopath)
Ostrow Institute for Pain Management
625 Madison Avenue, Suite 10A
New York, NY 10022
212-828-8265
www.ostrow.medem.com

Dr. Gottfried Kellerman (CEO of
Neuroscience Inc.)
Neuroscience, Inc.
373 280th Street
Osceola, WI 54020
888-342-7272
info@neuroscience.com

Dr. Stephen Koch (radiologist, clinical
instructor at Mt. Sinai School of
Medicine)
c/o Pulse Medical Imaging
4 Lyons Place
White Plains, NY 10601
914-325-4656
drkoch@kodean.com

LaVigne Organic Skin Care
#179, 205-329 North Road
Coquitlam, BC V3K 6Z8
Canada
866-931-6769
www.lavigneorganics.com

Dr. José Lladós-Comenge (endocrinologist)
P. O. Box 132

215

Stanfordville, NY 12581

845-868-7100 or 800-315-9305

www.drcomenge.com

Dr. Z. Paul Lorenc (plastic surgeon)

983 Park Avenue

New York, NY 10028

212-472-2900

www.lorenc.com

Dr. Marc Lowenberg (cosmetic dentist)

Lowenberg & Lituchy

230 Central Park South

New York, NY 10019

212-586-2890

www.lowenbergandlituchy.com

Dr. Jeffrey Mechanick (endocrinologist)

1192 Park Avenue

New York, NY 10128

212-831-2100

Miraval Spa and Resort

5000 E. Via Estancia Miraval

Catalina, AZ 85739

800-232-3969

www.miravalresort.com

Dr. Jeffrey Morrison (director of the

Morrison Center)

The Morrison Center

103 Fifth Avenue, 6th Floor

New York, NY 10003

212-989-9828

www.TheMorrisonCenter.com

www.DailyBenefit.com

Adina Niemerow (holistic chef)

adina@adinaniemerow.com

www.adinaniemerow.com

Dr. Nicholas Perricone

(dermatologist)

639 Research Parkway

Meriden, CT 06450

203-379-0726 or 888-823-7837

www.nvperriconemd.com

Gennero Sbarro (restaurateur)

Salute!

270 Madison Avenue (East 39th Street)

New York, NY 10016

212-213-3440

www.salutenyc.com

Dr. Erika Schwartz (physician, expert on

bioidentical hormones)

10 West 74th Street

New York, NY 10023

212-873-3420 or 866-373-7452

www.drerika.com

Oscar Smith (personal trainer, owner of

O-Diesel Studio)

O-Diesel Studio

39 White Street

New York, NY 10013
212-925-1466
www.odiesel.com

Warren & Tricomi (hairstylists)
15 West 57th Street, 4th floor
New York, NY 10019
212-262-8899
8327 Melrose Avenue
Los Angeles, CA 90069
323-651-4545
www.warrentricomi.com

Sheila Wormer (massage therapist)
Sheila.wormer@gmail.com

Dr. Lisa Zdinak
Precision Aesthetics
135 East 74th Street
New York, NY 10021
21-799-1411
drzdinak@precisionaesthetics.com
www.precisionaesthetics.com

Companies

Allergy Research Group
2300 North Loop Road
Alameda, CA 94502
800-545-9960
www.allergyresearchgroup.com

American Nutrition
735 North Park Street, Unit E

Castle Rock, CO 80104
800-454-3724
www.americannutrition.com

Apothecure
4001 McEwen Road, Suite 100
Dallas, TX 75244
800-969-6601
www.apothecure.com

Integrative Therapeutics Inc.
Customer Service Department
9 Monroe Parkway, Suite 250
Lake Oswego, OR 97035
800-931-1709
www.integrativeinc.com

Jarrow Formulas
1824 S. Robertson Boulevard
Los Angeles, CA 90035
800-726-0886
www.jarrow.com

Life Enhancement
P. O. Box 751390
Petaluma, CA 94975
800-LIFE-873
www.life-enhancement.com

Life Extension Foundation
1100 West Commercial Boulevard
Fort Lauderdale, FL 33309
800-544-4440
www.lef.org

217

Metagenics
166 Fernwood Avenue
Edison, NJ 08837
800-638-2848
www.metagenics.com

Nutraceutics
2217 NW 10th Terrace, Suite 404
Fort Lauderdale, FL 33309
800-391-0114
www.netraceutics.com

OPCPure
Max Bena Distributions
651 E. Alvarado Street
Pomona, CA 91767
877-410-ENERGY
www.opcpure.com

Phoenix Pharmaceuticals
800-988-1205
info@phoenixpeptide.com
www.phoenixpeptide.com

PhytoPharmica Inc.
825 Challenger Drive
Green Bay, WI 54311
800-376-7889

Pure Encapsulations
Pure Prescriptions Inc.

535 Encinitas Boulevard, Suite 118
Encinitas, CA 92024
800-860-9583
www.pureprescriptions.com

Source Naturals
19 Janis Way
Scotts Valley, CA 95066
800-815-2333
www.sourcenaturals.com

TriMedica
TriMedica International Inc.
1895 South Los Feliz
    Drive
Tempe, AZ 85281
800-800-8849
www.trimedica.com

Twinlab
150 Motor Parkway,
    Suite 210
Hauppauge, NY 11788
800-645-5626
www.twinlab.com

Xymogen Inc.
725 S. Kirkman Road
Orlando, FL 32811
800-647-6100
www.xymogen.com

INDEX

❧

225

MORE ADVICE FROM OZ GARCIA

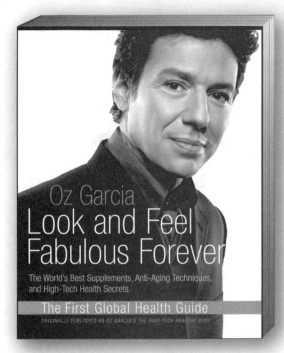

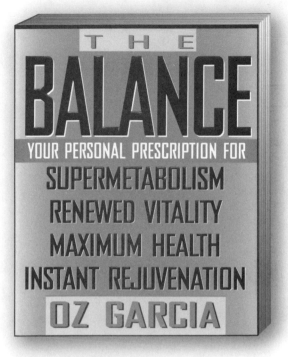

LOOK AND FEEL FABULOUS FOREVER
The World's Best Supplements, Anti-Aging Techniques, and High-Tech Health Secrets

ISBN 978-0-06-098890-6 (paperback)

Covering such diverse conditions and problems as thinning hair, diminished sexual function, poor muscle tone, vision problems, memory lapses, anxiety, weight gain, osteoporosis, and dental flaws, this comprehensive guide discusses the finest health supplements, procedures, products, techniques, and technology in the world today. No other book offers this kind of information on today's high-tech breakthroughs!

THE BALANCE
Your Personal Prescription for *Super Metabolism *Renewed Vitality *Maximum Health *Instant Rejuvenation

ISBN 978-0-06-098737-4 (paperback)

Do you have a fast metabolism? A slow metabolism? Something in between? Do you anger easily...or tend toward depression? What kinds of food do you crave? Your answers to these and other questions determine your metabolic profile and what types of foods and supplements will help you use your own natural resources to turn your body into a lean, vital, fat-burning machine—the state Oz calls *The Balance*.

Learn More • Do More • Live More

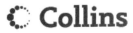 **Collins** *An Imprint of* HarperCollins*Publishers* www.harpercollins.com